Placentitis and Perinatal Infections

Vsevolod Zinserling • Andrey Kolobov
Sebastian Lucas

Placentitis and Perinatal Infections

Issues of Pathology and Pathogenesis

Springer

Vsevolod Zinserling
Institute of Experimental Medicine
Federal Almazov North-West Medical
Research
Saint Petersburg, Russia

Andrey Kolobov
Department of Pathology
Saint-Petersburg State University
Saint-Petersburg, Russia

Sebastian Lucas
Retired pathologist, previously at
Department of Cellular Pathology
St Thomas' Hospital
London, UK

ISBN 978-3-031-80552-3 ISBN 978-3-031-80553-0 (eBook)
https://doi.org/10.1007/978-3-031-80553-0

This Springer imprint is published by the registered company Springer Nature Switzerland AG
The registered company address is: Gewerbestrasse 11, 6330 Cham, Switzerland

Introduction

It is obvious that in order to reduce infant mortality and child disability, it is essential to develop preventive measures for the development of a number of diseases that most often act as their causes. Unfortunately, the level of diagnostic work, including pathological, varies significantly across certain regions and countries, which makes it impossible to assess the data of official world statistics on the causes of infant mortality as absolutely reliable. In United Kingdom, official statistics does not include infections as a cause of infant death. In addition, the figures provided usually relate to large groups of diseases, often entire classes of ICD. Nevertheless, it seems possible to note that the majority of cases of infant mortality included in the official statistics fall on "separate conditions of the perinatal period" and on congenital anomalies.

Without being able to comprehensively characterize the initial causes and etiology of these processes, it is safe to say that a significant portion of them may be associated with the infectious pathology of the placenta. More accurate representations can be obtained only with a detailed analysis of selected materials. According to St. Petersburg [1], a significant part of the observations with asphyxia, pneumopathy, congenital pneumonia, and sepsis is accompanied by a variety of intrauterine infections, which are able to contribute to their pathogenesis.

The placenta is a temporary organ that ensures the development and birth of a viable fetus. A normal placenta delivers oxygen, nutrients, and minerals to the fetus from the mother's blood by simple diffusion or active transport and cleavage and synthesis of substances at the trophoblast level. It produces steroid and polypeptide hormones and also performs a barrier function. This organ is an integral part of the complex mother–placenta–fetus system and ensures the existence and development of an embryo alien to the mother in terms of the antigenic structure. It is obvious that almost all aspects of both the intrauterine development of the embryo and fetus and the postnatal existence of a newborn (and sometimes an older child) directly or indirectly depend on the condition of the placenta.

Exceptionally great importance in modern medicine is attached to the problem of "hidden" urogenital infections. One can talk about the importance of both practical and theoretical aspects of this issue. In numerous literature on urogenital infections, the main attention is paid to the issues of diagnosis (mainly using PCR and ELISA) and treatment. Many other questions, including those related to the role of the placenta in intrauterine infection, are practically not considered at all.

Recently, no one has any doubts about the exceptionally great importance that intrauterine infections have in the pathology of childhood. In addition to the already well-studied severe forms of these diseases, which often cause fatal outcomes in the perinatal period, their other variants, characterized by a not so striking, but very long course, leading to a variety of somatic and neurological pathology, are beginning to attract increasing attention.

For many years, study of infectious perinatology has been carried out at the scientific school of A.V. Zinserling (1923–1995), which successfully researched infections of various localizations. Intrauterine infections and placentitis, primarily caused by various types of mycoplasmas, herpes viruses, and chlamydia, have been widely studied. The morphological changes caused by these pathogens have been described in detail for the first time in the world. It has been established that the changes caused by them are fundamentally the same as in other tissues and have diagnostic significance. A number of new priority facts have been identified, and the possible role of intrauterine infections in the occurrence of congenital malformations, premature birth, prematurity, and immaturity has been proven. Important data have been obtained on the nature of the lesion of the placenta and on the compensation processes occurring in it. The possibility of a tentative cytological diagnosis of mycoplasmosis, chlamydia, and herpes in smears from the cervix and urethra in women is substantiated, which allows, if there are clinical indications, to begin etiotropic treatment. In the 1990s, a system of urgent placental studies was developed and implemented to identify risk groups among newborns and mothers.

Despite the significant number of publications by A.V. Zinserling and his collaborators devoted to the problem of placentitis and intrauterine infections (largely in Russian), a number of issues remained insufficiently covered.

Numerous studies in recent decades have provided new information on the ultrastructure and immunohistochemistry of syncytiotrophoblast, cytotrophoblast, stroma cells, endothelium, and capillaries of villi and fetal membranes. However, information about infectious lesions of the placenta, given even in the most complete and authoritative manuals [2–4] are very brief and incomplete. Modern reviews devoted to intrauterine infections discuss all aspects of the problem except pathology [5].

We could not find reliable data on the frequency of all intrauterine infections based on screening laboratory and histological methods in different regions of the world.

The data on intrauterine infections in the latest edition of *The Potter's Manual* (2007) are largely based on data from previous years. Within the framework of the congresses of the European Society of Pathology and the Pediatric Pathology Society, little attention has been paid to infectious perinatology lately.

All this prompted us to summarize the available materials.

References

1. Zinserling VA, Melnikova VF. Perinatal infections: questions of pathogenesis, morphological diagnostics and clinic–pathological correlations. Practical manual. SPb: Elbi–SPb; 2002, 352p (in Russian).
2. Benirschke K, Burton GJ, Baergen RN. Pathology of the human placenta. 6th ed. Berlin: Springer; 2012, 941p.
3. Kay HH, Nelson DM, Wang Y. The placenta: from development to disease. 1st ed. Hoboken: Wiley-Blackwell; 2011, 360p. https://doi.org/10.1002/9781444393927.
4. Khong TY, Mooney EE, Nikkels PGJ, Morgan TK, Gordijn S. Pathology of the placenta: a practical guide. 1st ed. Switzerland: Springer Nature; 2019, 395p. https://doi.org/10.1007/978-3-319-97214-5.
5. Auriti C, De Rose DU, Santisi A, Martini L, Piersigilli F, Bersani I, Ronchetti MP, Caforio L. Pregnancy and viral infections: mechanisms of fetal damage, diagnosis and prevention of neonatal adverse outcomes from cytomegalovirus to SARS-CoV-2 and Zika virus. Biochim Biophys Acta Mol basis Dis. 2021;1867(10):166198. https://doi.org/10.1016/j.bbadis.2021.166198.

Contents

1 Morphogenesis of the Human Placenta

In the early stages of gestation, a number of key processes are consistently carried out that determine the further successful development of pregnancy: implantation, placentation, and the first wave of invasion of cytotrophoblastic cells [1, 2].

After fertilization and the formation of a zygote in the period of blastogenesis, a morula is formed as a result of the division of blastomeres. Approximately at the stage of 58 blastomeres, fluid appears inside the morula, a cavity (blastocoel) is formed, and the embryo turns into a blastocyst. In the blastocyst, the outer layer of cells is distinguished—the trophoblast, which gives rise to the placenta and membranes of the embryo, and the inner cell mass—the germinal nodule, or embryoblast, from which the fetus develops later [3] (Fig. 1.1).

From the seventh day, implantation begins—the introduction of the blastocyst into the uterine wall, in which the embryo is completely immersed in the uterine mucosa, and the mucosa fuses over the embryo (interstitial implantation) [3]. In turn, both the formation of a zygote and implantation are referred to as critical phases of embryogenesis, which predetermine the formation of the functions of the body and its systems at the next stage of development [1].

Trophoblast derivatives are villi. In the early stages of ontogenesis, the trophoblast forms protoplasmic outgrowths consisting of cytotrophoblast cells (primary villi). These villi do not have vessels, and the supply of nutrients and oxygen to the body of the embryo from the surrounding maternal blood occurs according to the laws of osmosis and diffusion. By the end of the 2nd week of pregnancy, secondary villi are formed: their basis is connective tissue, and the outer cover is represented by epithelium—syncytio—and cytotrophoblast. Both primary and secondary villi are evenly distributed over the surface of the ovum. As a result, a shell, the chorion, is formed around the embryo [2].

Later on, the villous chorion (chorion frondosum) is located mainly in the region of the implantation pole, and it is from it that the fetal part of the placenta develops—the chorionic plate and villi [2].

In the rest of the area, villous formations are reduced, which is why it is called the smooth chorion (chorion laeve). Remains of reduced villi remain in some parts of the smooth chorion [3].

From the 3rd week of intrauterine development, part of the mesenchymal cells of the stroma of secondary villi differentiates into cellular elements of the walls of blood capillaries (autochthonous angiogenesis) (Fig. 1.2). From this time, the period of placentation is considered to start, which lasts until the 12th week of pregnancy. At the same time, blood vessels grow from the side of the allantois. On average, on the 32nd day, the vessels of allantois are connected to the capillaries of the villi (Fig. 1.3). The villi turn into tertiary and blood circulation between the fetus and the placenta is established—fetoplacental circulation.

V. Zinserling et al., *Placentitis and Perinatal Infections*,
https://doi.org/10.1007/978-3-031-80553-0_1

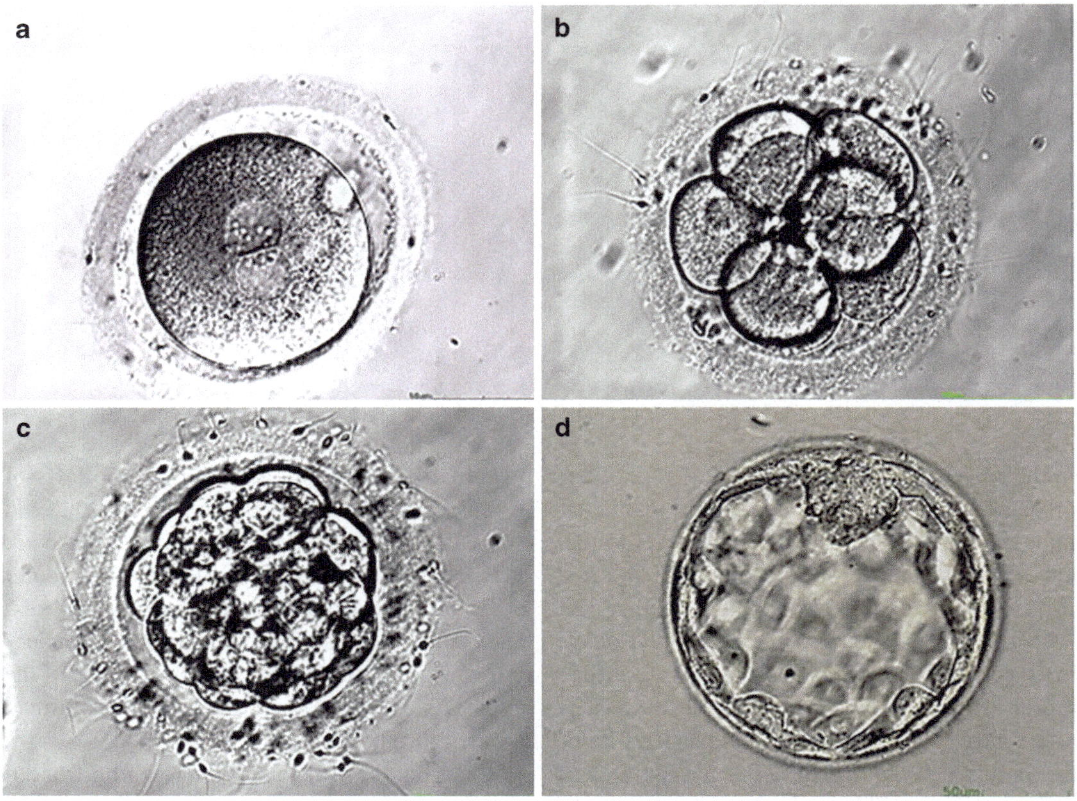

Fig. 1.1 Stages of development of the embryo in the period of blastogenesis. (**a**) Zygote, ×400; (**b**) 3–day–old embryo (seven blastomeres), ×400; (**c**) morula, ×400; (**d**) blastocyst, ×200

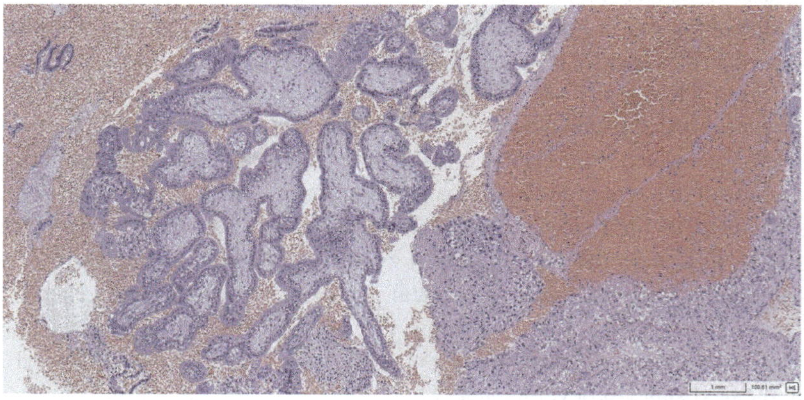

Fig. 1.2 Embryonal villi, 4 weeks of gestation, H&E, ×100

The precursor of all types of volli is of mesenchymal origine, which corresponds to the tertiary villi that occur during the early stages of placentation. As these villi grow and elongate during the first and second trimesters of pregnancy, they gradually differentiate first into immature intermediate and then into stem villi. The source of new generations of villi in the developing placenta is trophoblastic buds that appear on the surface of mesenchymal and immature intermediate villi. They form processes and turn into new branches of mesenchymal villi. The division of the villi is predominantly dichotomous in nature [4].

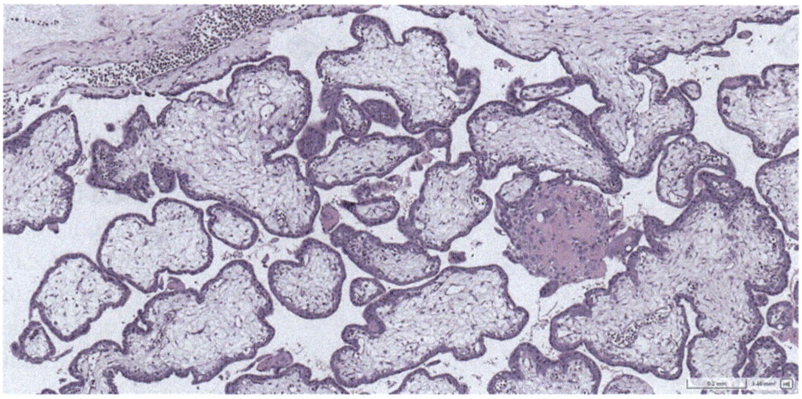

Fig. 1.3 Villous chorion, 6 weeks of gestation, H&E, ×200

Thus, after the 3rd week of pregnancy, most of the villi should contain blood vessels. The main frame of the villous tree is formed, which in the first half of pregnancy is represented by three types of villi: stem, intermediate immature, and mesenchymal. At the same time, during the period of placentation, large stem (supporting) villi with a diameter of 160 μm to 2 mm predominate. Their vascular network is represented by both fetal arteries and veins and capillaries. The mesenchyme of the stroma of the villi differentiates with the appearance in it of thin reticular fibers, fibroblast cells of varying degrees of maturity, and placental macrophages (Hofbauer cells: in Russian literature by certain reasons called Kashchenko-Hofbauer cells) [5]. Hofbauer cells are large (10–40 μm in diameter) rounded cells (Fig. 1.4). They are present in the chorionic villi throughout pregnancy, located in the zone of stromal channels and, in percentage terms, can be up to 40% of all non-trophoblastic cells of the villi [6].

Their population in the stroma of immature villi progressively increases until the 18th week of pregnancy, which corresponds to the period of maximum growth rate of the placenta [7]. In the third trimester of a physiologically proceeding pregnancy, the number of placental macrophages in the chorionic villi decreases [8].

CD14 is the most "universal" monocyte/macrophage marker. CD14+ macrophages isolated from at term human placentas are of both maternal (30%) and fetal origin (70%) [6]. Like macrophages in other organs, placental macrophages

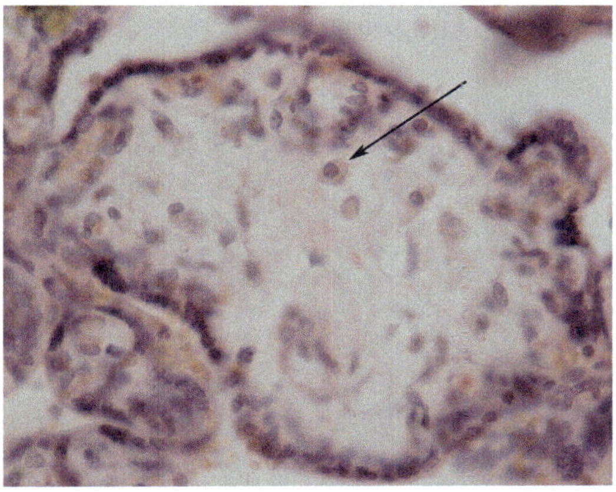

Fig. 1.4 Hofbauer cell (arrow), 22–23 weeks of gestation, H&E, ×400

carry this molecule on the cell membrane (Fig. 1.5).

When studying placental tissue or cells isolated from it, CD14 expression is considered as a sufficient criterion for belonging to macrophages [9, 10]. However, according to some authors, in the mature placenta, Hofbauer cells have the CD14low and even CD14– phenotype [11–13]. Placental macrophages also specifically express CD68 (macrosialin), CD136, and lectin [7]. There is an opinion about non-specific staining with CD68 as a macrophage marker, since its expression is found in other cell types, in particular, fibroblasts (Fig. 1.6) [14, 15].

In addition, Hofbauer cells express, although to a lower extent than other macrophages, CD4 and CCR5 [16–18].

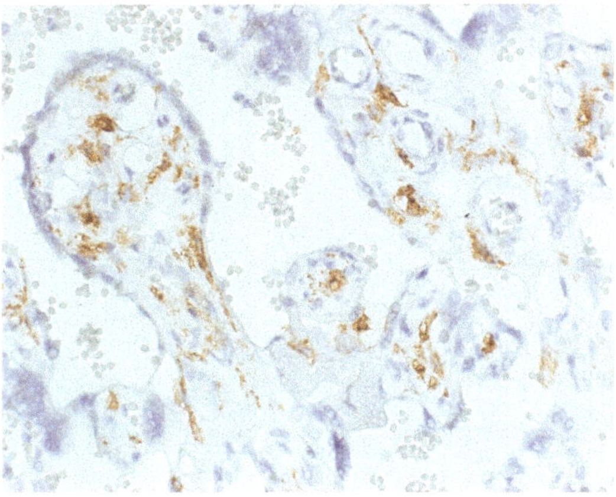

Fig. 1.5 Expression of CD14 in cells inside of villi in term placenta, IHC, ×400

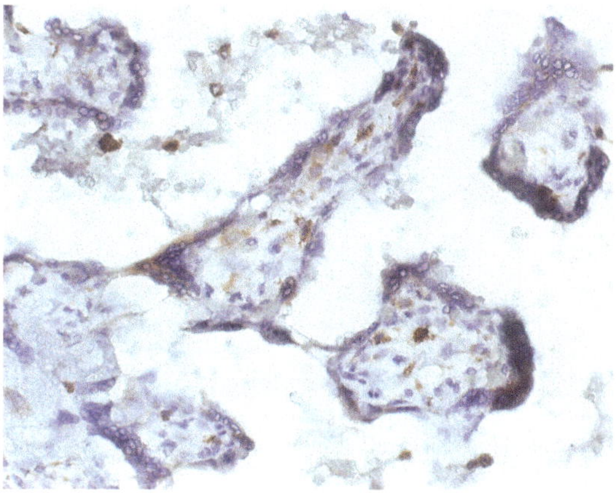

Fig. 1.6 Expression of CD68 by villi cells in term placenta, IHC, ×400

Immune tolerance may be mediated by DC–SIGN (+) dendritic cells of the decidua, especially in early pregnancy [19]. DC–SIGN (dendritic cell-specific ICAM-grabbing non-integrin, CD209) interacts with ICAM-3 T-lymphocytes [20]. DC–SIGN was detected on the surface of specialized placental macrophages [21]. In turn, Mummidi et al. [20] noted the presence of the DC–SIGN2 gene, while the original gene is designated DC–SIGN1. The authors revealed the expression of DC–SIGN1 mRNA in THP-1 monocytic cells, peripheral blood mononuclear cells, placenta, in particular, on endothelial cells and CCR5-positive placental macrophages [20, 21].

At the 5th to 6th week of pregnancy, 2/3 of the epithelial layer of villi is formed by syncytiotrophoblast. In the period from 4th to 6th, and then from the 8th to the 12th week of intrauterine development, there is a wave-like increase in maternal blood flow to the placenta. This happens due to the activity of the cytotrophoblast of cell columns. Freely located islets of trophoblastic epithelium continue to destroy endometrial tissues, which occurs due to their proliferation and enzymatic activity both in the endometrial stroma (interstitial trophoblast) and inside the endometrial vessels (intravascular trophoblast). As a result, the endometrial segments of the spiral arteries of the endometrium are opened, after which a constant uteroplacental blood flow is established. This stage of placentation is also attributed to the critical phases of human embryogenesis [1].

The chorionic epithelium, or trophoblast, in the early stages of development is represented by cytotrophoblast—a single-layer epithelium with oval nuclei. These cells reproduce by mitosis. Of these, a syncytiotrophoblast develops—a multinuclear structure covering the reducing cytotrophoblast. This structure results from the fusion and differentiation of mitotically active cytotrophoblast cells. With the course of pregnancy, the trophoblast becomes single-layered and continuous.

Genes of human endogenous retroviruses (HERVs family) are involved in the regulation of intercellular fusion of cytotrophoblast elements and formation of syncytiotrophoblast, which are remnants of ancestral retroviruses fixed in human DNA. The existence of HERVs became known in the second half of the twentieth century, but their representation in the human genome and functions have not been elucidated until recently. In subsequent years, more than 30 new families were identified [22].

Syncytin-1 (ERVWE1—Endogenous Retroviral family W, Env(C7), member 1) was the first protein from the HERV family for which a role in placental cell fusion was proven. Under physiological conditions, syncytin-1 is expressed exclusively in trophoblast cells—both cyto- and (to a greater extent) syncytiotrophoblast [23, 24].

In turn, the expression of syncytin-1 can activate pro-inflammatory cytokines (IL-β) and iNOS. Through the phenomenon of receptor interference, syncytin-1 protects host cells from exogenous retroviruses [22].

Syncytin-1, together with TGF-β1 or TGF-β3, and also through the mechanism of delaying apoptosis of syncytiotrophoblast, is involved in the regulation of the proliferation of villous trophoblast and cytotrophoblast of cell columns. This anti-apoptotic function is mediated by Bcl-2 [25]. Dai et al. [26] showed that apoptotic changes in placental cells under conditions of oxygen starvation can be regulated by hypoxia-inducible factors—HIF-la, HIF-2a, and HIF-1β.

In addition, the regulator of apoptosis is the Fas system—Fas ligand (FasL) and its Fas receptor. In ensuring fetal tolerance to maternal HIV infection is reported that Fas receptor, interacting with FasL, a transmembrane-T-killer protein, is activated ad trigger the death program of an HIV-infected cell [27, 28].

Syncytin-2, belonging to the endogenous retrovirus group FRD, is also actively involved in the formation of trophoblast cells symplasts [29, 30]. Also, syncytin-2 is characterized by immunosuppressive activity, and, according to M. Mangeney et al. [30], it is higher than that of syncytin-1.

U.Kämmerer et al. [31] studied the endogenous retrovirus HERV-K in their work. Thus, it was shown that the TM protein HERV-K is expressed exclusively by cytotrophoblast elements, both villous and peripheral. The authors also believe that HERV-K is actively involved in the immune defense of the fetus.

Intercellular cooperation is also essential. There is evidence that the activation of NK cells occurs under the influence of interferon produced by the trophoblast. However, the widespread antigens of the HLA group—A, B, functionally closely related to NK cells are not expressed on the surface of the trophoblast. HLA-G is considered as the most important antigen of this localization. In addition, there are receptors for the Fc fragment of immunoglobulin G on the membranes of syncytiotrophoblast [1].

Growth, differentiation, invasion, and migration of the trophoblast are regulated, in particular, by placenta growth factor (PlGF), insulin-like growth factor ILGF, endothelial vascular growth factor VEGF (including isoforms VEGF-A VEGF-B, VEGF-C, VEGF-D, VEGF-E) and transforming growth factor TGF-β2 [32–35].

In early pregnancy, angiogenesis by branching predominates. It proceeds under hypoxic conditions and is controlled by VEGF through VEGFR-2 [35, 36]. Stimulation of the VEGFR-2 receptor leads to the inhibition of angiogenesis and the development of endothelial dysfunction. So, the content of VEGFR-2, angiogenin, which is a mediator between VEGF and VEGFR-2, and angiopoietin-2, which is a mediator between VEGF and VEGFR-1, increases with placental insufficiency. At later stages, angiogenesis proceeds without branching with sufficient oxygen supply to tissues and is controlled by PlGF through VEGFR-1. The degree of P1GF expression increases with an increase in the partial pressure of oxygen and decreases with its decrease. At the same time, VEGF expression is maximally high at low oxygen partial pressure [36].

Fibroblast growth factors (FGFs) are also referred to as proangiogenic substances. The FGF family currently has nine members. Representatives of the FGF–family FGF-1 (acid fibroblast growth factor—aFGF) and FGF-2 (basic fibroblast growth factor—bFGF) are products of different genes and have up to 53.0% amino acid homology. Seven FGF subfamilies have been defined based on their sequence homology and function. These FGF subfamilies can also be divided into two general groups, the canonical FGFs comprising paracrine or autocrine-acting FGF1-10, FGF16-18, FGF20, and FGF22 and the endocrine-acting FGFs, FGF15 (mouse)/FGF19 (human), FGF21, and FGF23; and the non-canonical FGFs comprising FGF11-14 [37]. bFGF controls various stages of angiogenesis, promotes the survival of endothelial cells and their protection from apoptosis, which is also associated with an increase in Bcl-2 expression. FGF stimulates DNA synthesis and division of various cells of mesenchymal origin, in particular smooth muscle cells and endotheliocytes [37]. Both of these cell types are involved in the formation of vascular walls. bFGF is able to act intracellularly as a proliferation activator. In vitro studies have found the possibility of synergism between VEGF and bFGF in the induction of angiogenesis [34]. Thrombospondin is one of the main inhibitors of angiogenesis, affecting the adhesion and growth of endothelial cells and competing with FGF for cell-cell binding [38].

Placental coordination begins with the cells that comprise the maternal–fetal interface, termed the placental barrier, that receive signals from both maternal and fetal circulation. Placental barrier, in a functional sense, it is regarded as the equivalent of the diffusion properties of the placenta, and in a narrow sense, as the ultrastructural part of the vasculosyncytial membrane. Electron microscopic examination showed that the membrane has seven layers—syncytiotrophoblast, light space, two basement membranes of trophoblast with collagen tissue between them, basement membrane of the endothelium of the germinal capillary, endothelium. The ultrastructural and molecular structure of the placental barrier is maximally adapted for intensive diffusion processes [39].

Damage to the placental barrier creates the prerequisites for infection of the intrauterine developing fetus.

References

1. Kay HH, Nelson DM, Wang Y. The placenta: from development to disease. 1st ed. Hoboken: Wiley-Blackwell; 2011, 360p. https://doi.org/10.1002/9781444393927.
2. Kojima J, Ono M, Kuji N, Nishi H. Human chorionic villous differentiation and placental development. Int J Mol Sci. 2022;23(14):8003. https://doi.org/10.3390/ijms23148003.
3. Benirschke K, Burton GJ, Baergen RN. Pathology of the human placenta. 6th ed. Berlin: Springer; 2012, 941p.
4. Wang Y, Zhao S. Vascular biology of the placenta. San Rafael: Morgan & Claypool Life Sciences; 2010, 98p. https://doi.org/10.4199/C00016ED1V01Y201008ISP009.
5. Baergen RN. Manual of Benirschke and Kaufmann's pathology of the human placenta. Berlin: Springer; 2005, 504p.
6. Mezouar S, Katsogiannou M, Amara AB, Bretelle F, Mege JL. Placental macrophages: origin, heterogeneity, function and role in pregnancy-associated infections. Placenta. 2021;103:94–103. https://doi.org/10.1016/j.placenta.2020.10.017.
7. Ingman K, Cookson VJ, Jones CJ, Aplin JD. Characterisation of Hofbauer cells in first and second trimester placenta: incidence, phenotype, survival in vitro and motility. Placenta. 2010;31:535–44. https://doi.org/10.1016/j.placenta.2010.03.003.
8. Vinnars MT, Rindsjö E, Ghazi S, Sundberg A, Papadogiannakis N. The number of CD68(+) (Hofbauer) cells is decreased in placentas with chorioamnionitis and with advancing gestational age. Pediatr Dev Pathol. 2010;13(4):300–4. https://doi.org/10.2350/09-03-0632-OA.1.
9. Cupurdija K, Azzola D, Hainz U, et al. Macrophages of human first trimester decidua express markers associated to alternative activation. Am J Reprod Immunol. 2004;51(2):117–22. https://doi.org/10.1046/j.8755-8920.2003.00128.x.
10. Phillips TA, Ni J, Hunt JS. Death-inducing tumour necrosis factor (TNF) superfamily ligands and receptors are transcribed in human placentae, cytotrophoblasts, placental macrophages and placental cell lines. Placenta. 2001;22(8–9):663–72. https://doi.org/10.1053/plac.2001.0703.
11. Blaschitz A, Weiss U, Dohr G, Desoye G. Antibody reaction patterns in first trimester placenta: implications for trophoblast isolation and purity screening. Placenta. 2000;21(7):733–41. https://doi.org/10.1053/plac.2000.0559.
12. Kim J-S, Romero R, Kim MR, Kim YM, Friel L, Espinoza J, Kim CJ. Involvement of Hofbauer cells and maternal T cells in villitis of unknown aetiology. Histopathology. 2008;52(4):457–64. https://doi.org/10.1111/j.1365-2559.2008.02964.x.
13. McIntire RH, Petroff MG, Phillips TA, Hunt JS. In vitro models for studying human uterine and placental macrophages. Methods Mol Med. 2006;122:123–48. https://doi.org/10.1385/1-59259-989-3:123.
14. Kunisch E, Fuhrmann R, Roth A, Winter R, Lungershausen W, Kinne R. Macrophage specificity of three anti-CD68 monoclonal antibodies (KP1, EBM11, and PGM1) widely used for immunohistochemistry and flow cytometry. Ann Rheum Dis. 2004;63(7):774–84. https://doi.org/10.1136/ard.2003.013029.
15. Pilling D, Fan T, Huang D, Kaul B, Gomer RH. Identification of markers that distinguish monocyte-derived fibrocytes from monocytes, macrophages, and fibroblasts. PLoS One. 2009;4(10):e7475. https://doi.org/10.1371/journal.pone.0007475.
16. García K, García V, Laspiur JP, Duan F, Meléndez LM. Characterization of the placental macrophage secretome: implications for antiviral activity. Placenta. 2009;30(2):149–55. https://doi.org/10.1016/j.placenta.2008.10.014.

17. García-Crespo K, Cadilla C, Skolasky R, Meléndez LM. Restricted HIV-1 replication in placental macrophages is caused by inefficient viral transcription. J Leukoc Biol. 2010;87(4):633–6. https://doi.org/10.1189/jlb.0809556.
18. Melendez J, García V, Sánchez E, Delgado R, Torres G, Meléndez-Guerrero LM. Is decreased HIV-1 infectivity of placental macrophages caused by high levels of beta-chemokines? Cell Mol Biol (Noisy-le-grand). 2001;47:Online Pub OL51–59.
19. Geijtenbeek T, Kwon DS, Torensma R, van Vliet SJ, et al. DC-SIGN, a dendritic cell-specific HIV-1-binding protein that enhances trans-infection of T cells. Cell. 2000;100(5):587–97. https://doi.org/10.1016/s0092-8674(00)80694-7.
20. Mummidi S, Catano G, Lam L, Hoefle A, Telles V, Begum K, Jimenez F, Ahuja SS, Ahuja SK. Extensive repertoire of membrane-bound and soluble dendritic cell-specific ICAM-3-grabbing nonintegrin 1 (DC-SIGN1) and DC-SIGN2 isoforms. Inter-individual variation in expression of DC-SIGN transcripts. J Biol Chem. 2001;276(35):33196–212. https://doi.org/10.1074/jbc.M009807200.
21. Soilleux EJ, Morris LS, Rushbrook S, Lee B, Coleman N. Expression of human immunodeficiency virus (HIV)-binding lectin DC-SIGNR: consequences for HIV infection and immunity. Hum Pathol. 2002;33(6):652–9. https://doi.org/10.1053/hupa.2002.124036.
22. van der Kuyl AC. HIV infection and HERV expression: a review. Retrovirology. 2012;9:6. https://doi.org/10.1186/1742-4690-9-6.
23. Noorali S, Rotar IC, Lewis C, Pestaner JP, Pace DG, Sison A, Bagasra O. Role of HERV-W syncytin-1 in placentation and maintenance of human pregnancy. Appl Immunohistochem Mol Morphol. 2009;17(4):319–28. https://doi.org/10.1097/PAI.0b013e31819640f9.
24. Rote NS, Chakrabarti S, Stetzer BP. The role of human endogenous retroviruses in trophoblast differentiation and placental development. Placenta. 2004;25(8–9):673–83. https://doi.org/10.1016/j.placenta.2004.02.008.
25. Forbes K, Westwood M. Maternal growth factor regulation of human placental development and fetal growth. J Endocrinol. 2010;207(1):1–16. https://doi.org/10.1677/JOE-10-0174.
26. Dai SY, Kanenishi K, Ueno M, Sakamoto H, Hata T. Hypoxia-inducible factor-2alpha is involved in enhanced apoptosis in the placenta from pregnancies with fetal growth restriction. Pathol Int. 2004;54(11):843–9. https://doi.org/10.1111/j.1440-1827.2004.01750.x.
27. Laforge M, Campillo-Gimenez L, Monceaux V, Cumont M-C, Hurtrel B, Corbeil J, Zaunders J, Elbim C, Estaquier J. HIV/SIV infection primes monocytes and dendritic cells for apoptosis. PLoS Pathog. 2011;7(6):e1002087. https://doi.org/10.1371/journal.ppat.1002087.
28. Lee CL, Chiu PC, Lam KK, Siu S-O, Chu IK, Koistinen R, Koistinen H, Seppälä M, Lee K-F, Yeung WS. Differential actions of glycodelin-A on Th-1 and Th-2 cells: a paracrine mechanism that could produce the Th-2 dominant environment during pregnancy. Hum Reprod. 2011;26(3):517–26. https://doi.org/10.1093/humrep/deq381.
29. Chen CP, Chen LF, Yang SR, Chen CY, Ko CC, Chang GD, Chen H. Functional characterization of the human placental fusogenic membrane protein syncytin 2. Biol Reprod. 2008;79(5):815–23. https://doi.org/10.1095/biolreprod.108.069765.
30. Mangeney M, Renard M, Schlecht-Louf G, Bouallaga I, Heidmann O, Letzelter C, Richaud A, Ducos B, Heidmann T. Placental syncytins: genetic disjunction between the fusogenic and immunosuppressive activity of retroviral envelope proteins. Proc Natl Acad Sci USA. 2007;104(51):20534–9. https://doi.org/10.1073/pnas.0707873105.
31. Kämmerer U, Germeyer A, Stengel S, Kapp M, Denner J. Human endogenous retrovirus K (HERV-K) is expressed in villous and cytotrophoblast of cell columns cells of the human placenta. J Reprod Immunol. 2011;91(1–2):1–8. https://doi.org/10.1016/j.jri.2011.06.102.
32. Bhattacharjee J, Mohammad S, Goudreau AD, Adamo KB. Physical activity differentially regulates VEGF, PlGF, and their receptors in the human placenta. Physiol Rep. 2021;9(2):e14710. https://doi.org/10.14814/phy2.14710.
33. Li X, Eriksson U. Novel VEGF family members: VEGF-B, VEGF-C and VEGF-D. Int J Biochem Cell Biol. 2001;33(4):421–6. https://doi.org/10.1016/s1357-2725(01)00027-9.
34. Lymboussaki A, Olofsson B, Eriksson U, Alitalo K. Vascular endothelial growth factor (VEGF) and VEGF-C show overlapping binding sites in embryonic endothelia and distinct sites in differentiated adult endothelia. Circ Res. 1999;85(11):992–9. https://doi.org/10.1161/01.res.85.11.992.
35. Nagy JA, Dvorak AM, Dvorak HF. VEGF-A(164/165) and PlGF: roles in angiogenesis and arteriogenesis. Trends Cardiovasc Med. 2003;13(5):169–75. https://doi.org/10.1016/s1050-1738(03)00056-2.
36. Regnault TR, Orbus RJ, de Vrijer B, Davidsen ML, Galan HL, Wilkening RB, Anthony RV. Placental expression of VEGF, PlGF and their receptors in a model of placental insufficiency-intrauterine growth restriction (PI-IUGR). Placenta. 2002;23(2–3):132–44. https://doi.org/10.1053/plac.2001.0757.
37. Li X, Wang C, Xiao J, McKeehan WL, Wang F. Fibroblast growth factors, old kids on the new block. Semin Cell Dev Biol. 2016;53:155–67. https://doi.org/10.1016/j.semcdb.2015.12.014.
38. Edwards AK, van den Heuvel MJ, Wessels JM, LaMarre J, Croy BA, Tayade C. Expression of angiogenic basic fibroblast growth factor, platelet derived growth factor, thrombospondin-1 and their

receptors at the porcine maternal-fetal interface. Reprod Biol Endocrinol. 2011;9:5. https://doi.org/10.1186/1477-7827-9-5.

39. Arumugasaamy N, Rock KD, Kuo C-Y, Bale TL, Fisher JP. Microphysiological systems of the placental barrier. Adv Drug Deliv Rev. 2020;161–162:161–75. https://doi.org/10.1016/j.addr.2020.08.010.

2 The Concept of Placental Insufficiency

Currently, placental insufficiency is considered to be a syndrome caused by structural changes in it and characterized by the inability of the placenta to maintain an adequate exchange between the mother and fetus. Placental insufficiency occurs when the placenta fails to provide the fetus sufficient nutrients and secreted factors. A fundamentally important issue is the attitude to placental insufficiency as an independent symptom complex accompanying the underlying pathological condition. Functional failure of the placenta is the main cause of intrauterine hypoxia, fetal growth retardation, its damage during childbirth [1, 2].

According to the timing of occurrence, primary (up to 16 weeks of pregnancy) and secondary placental insufficiency are distinguished.

Primary placental insufficiency is one of the main causes of non-developing pregnancy of the first trimester and spontaneous abortion [3]. Morphological criteria for primary placental insufficiency are the insufficiency of cytotrophoblast of cell columns invasion into the spiral arteries of the placental bed; rheological disorders; pathological immaturity of villi; disturbance of the blood perfusion in the villi; lesion of the placental barrier; dysfunction of hormone production [4, 5].

The following variants of the functional state of the placenta can be noted:

- compensated state (placenta without pathology);
- acute placental insufficiency;
- chronic compensated insufficiency;
- chronic subcompensated insufficiency (both with and without intrauterine growth retardation);
- chronic decompensated insufficiency.

In the compensated placenta, mature terminal villi with 3–5 capillaries prevailed, villi with vasculosyncytial membranes accounted for at least 50%, active syncytial nodules of small and medium sizes were found in at least 40% of terminal villi. Involutive changes were mild.

Acute placental insufficiency is observed, as a rule, with the pathology of the labor. Morphological signs of acute placental insufficiency are violations of the uteroplacental circulation. The placenta blood supply is increased, its color on the cut is dark red or violet red, large hematomas are visible on the maternal surface and under the amnion. Microscopic examination reveals diffuse hyperemia of the villous chorion (Fig. 2.1).

In chronic compensated placental insufficiency, the maturity of the villous chorion generally corresponded to the gestational age, more than 50% of the villi were with excessive vascularization. Active syncytial nodules of medium and large size predomitated. Involutive changes were expressed moderately, mainly due to the deposition of fibrinoid in the subchorial intervillous space (Fig. 2.2).

V. Zinserling et al., *Placentitis and Perinatal Infections*,
https://doi.org/10.1007/978-3-031-80553-0_2

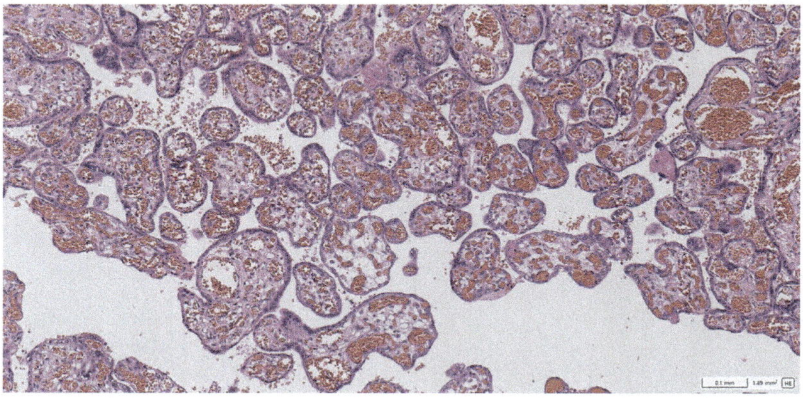

Fig. 2.1 Morphological signs of acute placental insufficiency: dilated full-blooded vessels of intermediate and terminal villi, 38 weeks of gestation, H&E, ×100

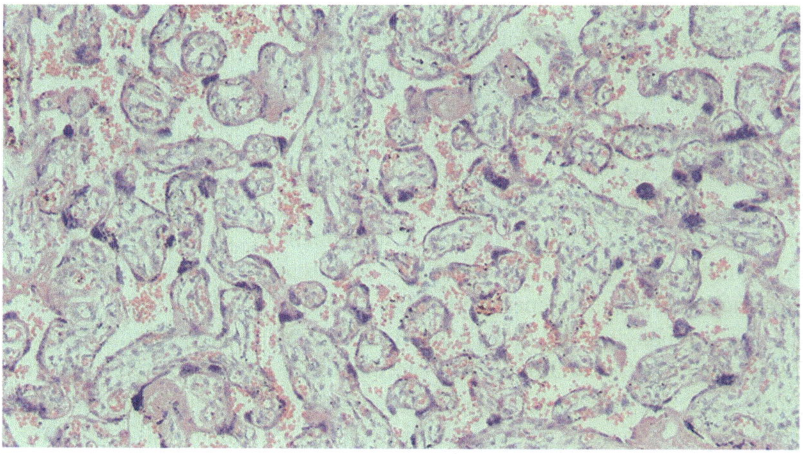

Fig. 2.2 Morphological signs of chronic compensated placental insufficiency: large syncytial nodules, moderate fibrinoid deposits in the intervillous space, 40 weeks of gestation, H&E, ×100

Chronic subcompensated placental insufficiency is characterized by pathological immaturity of the placenta, which is expressed in the dissociated development of the villous chorion, involutive processes, and circulatory disorders (Fig. 2.3).

The term “immaturity” is applied to placentas from 36 weeks of gestation [6]. The criterion for immaturity of villi (synonyms: delayed maturation of villi, maturation defect) is a small amount of vasculosyncytial membranes in comparison with mature villi, which are characterized by an increasing number of capillaries and the formation of vasculosyncytial membranes [7]. Immature for a gestational age of 36 weeks or more are placentas with predominant villi of an intermediate type—a relatively large diameter, with small vessels and abundant stroma, a trophoblast of uniform thickness, devoid of vasculosyncytial membranes and syncytial nodes. The variant, designated in the literature as premature maturation, is characterized by a significant decrease in the number of intermediate branches. It is important to note that the number of undifferentiated intermediate villi during premature maturation is very low, despite the fact that the gestation period for this variant is 31–32 weeks (Fig. 2.4).

So, in chronic decompensated insufficiency, a pronounced pathological immaturity of the villous chorion was noted—the presence of embryonic or immature intermediate villi, chaotic branching of the villi, involutive processes with poorly developed compensatory-adaptive reactions (both cellular—involutive, including calcified syncytial nodules, and vascular—reduction of the vascular bed and the presence of fields of chaotically sclerosed villi) (Fig. 2.5).

Placental insufficiency typically associated with abnormalities of perfusion which were

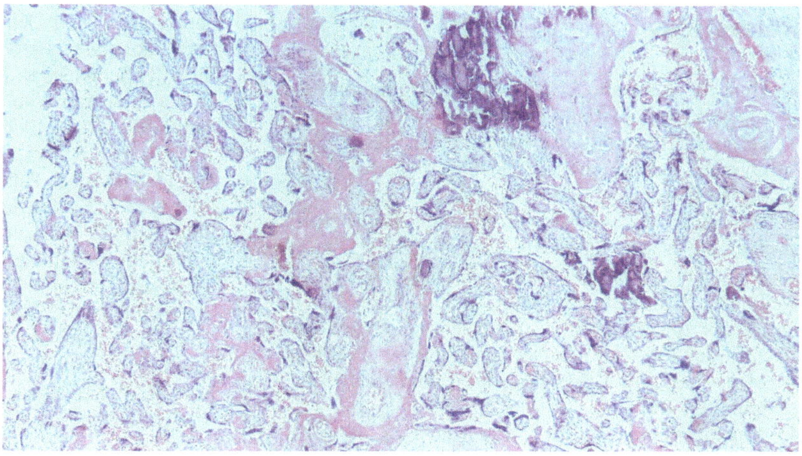

Fig. 2.3 Morphological signs of chronic subcompensated insufficiency of the placenta: impaired branching of the villous chorion with a predominance of intermediate villi, deposition of fibrinoid in the intervillous space, calcifies, 38 weeks of gestation, H&E, ×50

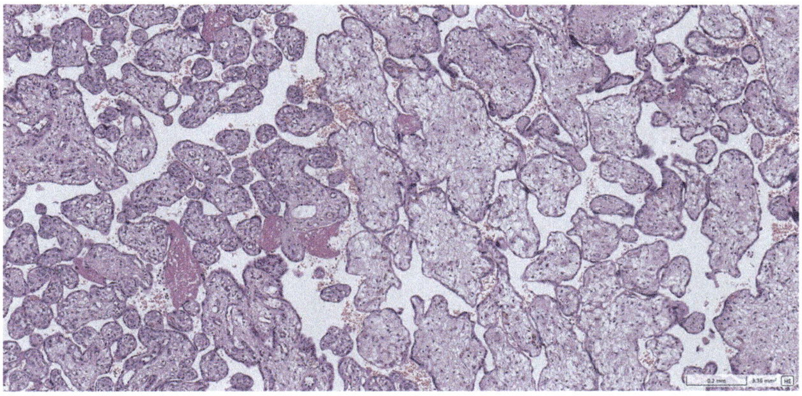

Fig. 2.4 Undifferentiated intermediate villi, 36 weeks of gestation, H&E, ×50

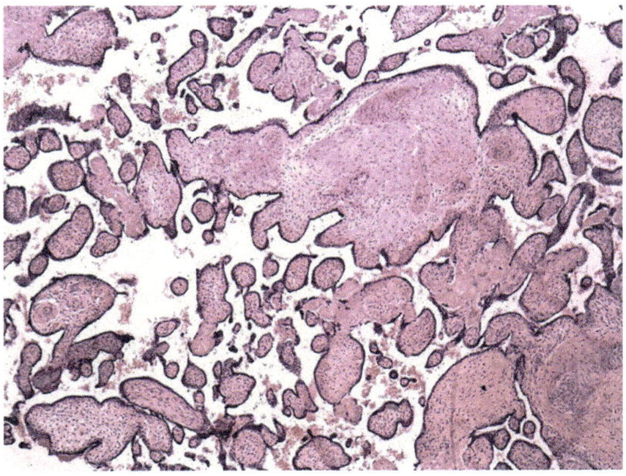

Fig. 2.5 The chaotically sclerosed villi, fibrinoid deposits in the intervillous space, 32 weeks of gestation, H&E, ×50

either fetal or maternal in origin. These malperfusive conditions result from a variety of processes including underlying maternal diseases (hypertensive diseases of pregnancy, diabetes, and maternal coagulopathies), fetal diseases (fetal coagulopathies, umbilical cord accidents, abnormal placental development, and implantation), environmental exposures (cigarette smoking), abruptions, and placental conditions such as maternal floor infarcts, massive perivillous fibrin deposition, villitis of unknown etiology, failure of physiological conversion of decidual arteries, and others [1]. Infections caused by TORCH agents typically do not produce placental insufficiency but instead exert their effects on the fetus after passing through the maternal–fetal interface at the placenta, entering the fetal bloodstream, reaching and directly infecting fetal organs [8].

References

1. Hunt K, Kennedy SH, Vatish M. Definitions and reporting of placental insufficiency in biomedical journals: a review of the literature. Eur J Obstet Gynecol Reprod Biol. 2016;205:146–9. https://doi.org/10.1016/j.ejogrb.2016.08.029.
2. Wardinger JE, Ambati S. Placental insufficiency. Treasure Island: StatPearls Publishing; 2022. http://www.ncbi.nlm.nih.gov/books/NBK563171/.
3. Jaiman S, Romero R, Bhatti G, Jung E, et al. The role of the placenta in spontaneous preterm labor and delivery with intact membranes. J Perinat Med. 2022;50(5):553–66. https://doi.org/10.1515/jpm-2021-0681.
4. Arumugasaamy N, Rock KD, Kuo C-Y, Bale TL, Fisher JP. Microphysiological systems of the placental barrier. Adv Drug Deliv Rev. 2020;161–162:161–75. https://doi.org/10.1016/j.addr.2020.08.010.
5. Silva JF, Serakides R. Intrauterine trophoblast migration: a comparative view of humans and rodents. Cell Adhes Migr. 2016;10(1–2):88–110. https://doi.org/10.1080/19336918.2015.1120397.
6. Fox H, Sebire NJ. Pathology of the placenta. 3rd ed. Philadelphia: Saunders, Elsevier; 2007, 574p.
7. Stallmach T, Hebisch G. Placental pathology: its impact on explaining prenatal and perinatal death. Virchows Arch. 2004;445(1):9–16. https://doi.org/10.1007/s00428-004-1032-2.
8. Megli CJ, Coyne CB. Infections at the maternal-fetal interface: an overview of pathogenesis and defence. Nat Rev Microbiol. 2022;20:67–82. https://doi.org/10.1038/s41579-021-00610-y.

3 General Principles and Methods of Morphological Diagnostics of Perinatal Infectious Pathology

The standardizing gross examination and histologic sampling of the placentas is carried out in according to Khong et al. [1].

Placental weight: Description of the placenta should include the placental weight trimmed of extraplacental membranes and umbilical cord, and notation of whether the placenta was fresh or fixed when measured. Any prior sampling of the placental parenchyma should also be documented. Any disruption of the basal plate should be noted. The placental weight is a surrogate for placental function, and fetoplacental weight ratio has been suggested as a possible indicator of adequacy of placental reserve capacity in fetal growth restriction. Where possible, contemporary placental weight standards derived from the respective local or similar population should be used.

Placental disk dimensions: Description of the placenta should include the measurement of the placenta in three dimensions: the maximal linear dimension (length), the greatest dimension of the axis perpendicular to this linear measurement (width), and the mural minimal and maximal thickness (Figs. 3.1 and 3.2). There is some evidence to suggest that shape and size of the placenta are factors that may be statistically associated with pregnancy complications (fetal growth restriction, reduced fetal movements) and an individual's long-term health. Measuring the placental dimensions will also allow further refinement of determining the functional reserve of the placenta by correlation of size of any lesions with the overall dimensions of the placenta.

Description of umbilical cord: It should include the average diameter of the cord; length; site of insertion in relation to the center/margin of the placenta, determined by measuring the distance between the insertion site and the nearest placental margin; the presence of strictures; and whether the cord appears to be hypocoiled or hypercoiled (Fig. 3.3).

Segmental or localized areas of hypercoiling should be recorded. Direction of coiling (handedness) should be noted if possible. Thin umbilical cords are associated with fetal growth restriction, whereas thick cords are associated with maternal diabetes and with fetal hydrops. Excessively long and short cords can be associated with adverse outcomes. Marginal (<1 cm from the nearest margin) and velamentous insertions, but not peripheral (<3 cm from the nearest margin) insertions, are associated with an increased risk of adverse pregnancy outcomes, including preterm delivery. Hypocoiling (<1 coil per 10 cm) and hypercoiling (>3 coils per 10 cm) may be associated with adverse outcomes in some cases. Opinion was divided about the best way to assess coiling, especially because cords are often incompletely submitted. Because not all of the cord may be received and because the significance of a localized site or segmental sites of hypercoiling is unclear, it was felt that such a nonuniform

V. Zinserling et al., *Placentitis and Perinatal Infections*,
https://doi.org/10.1007/978-3-031-80553-0_3

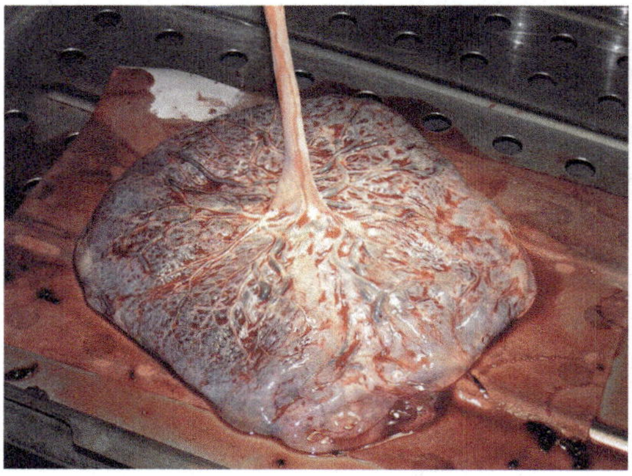

Fig. 3.1 Placental disk (fetal surface) and umbilical cord, term delivery

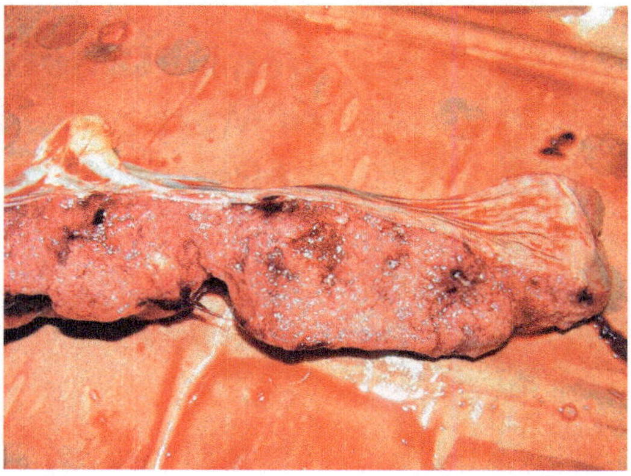

Fig. 3.2 Placental section for measurement thickness

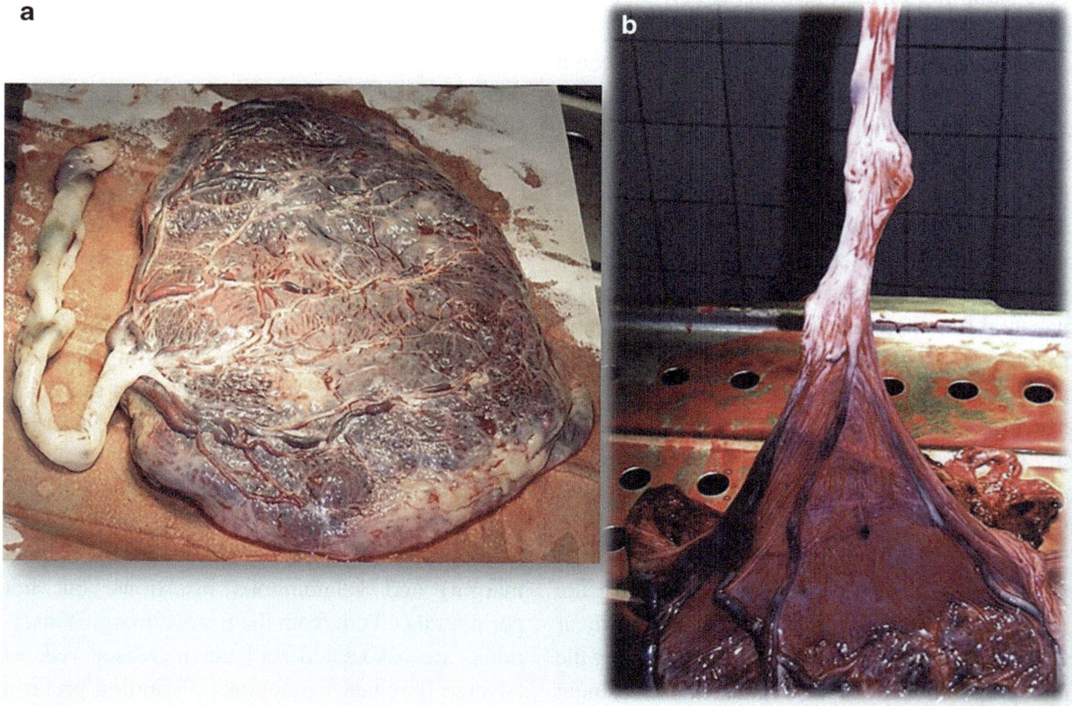

Fig. 3.3 Marginal (**a**) and velamentous (**b**) insertions of the umbilical cord

finding should be recorded until there was clarity regarding its significance. However, deep grooves between coils in hypercoiled cords have been associated with stillbirth and should be reported. Left twist, defined as diagonal seams running from upper left to lower right, is most common. The clinical significance of left versus right twist remains unclear, but it may useful to document this on a research basis.

Description of fetal membranes should include the color/opacity and completeness. Recording the shortest distance between the site of rupture to the placental edge may be useful in some cases of placenta previa if the rupture was

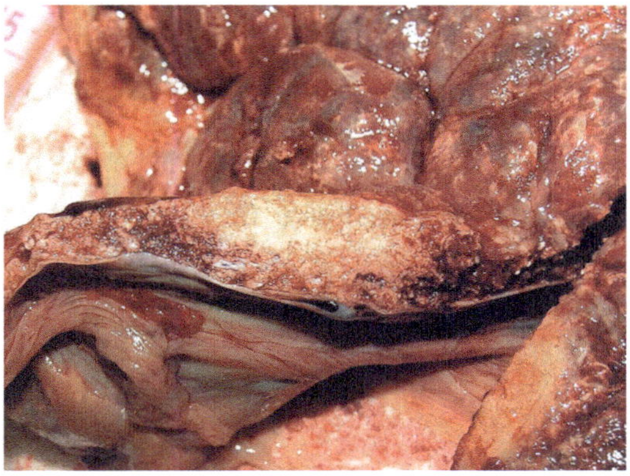

Fig. 3.4 Placental infarct

at the edge, but the group was divided on this recommendation. If circumvallate or circummarginate, the percentage of the circumference involved should be noted. Circumvallation may be associated with bleeding in early pregnancy and may show iron deposition in the membranes, sometimes with a yellow-brown or brown discoloration. Iron and meconium pigments are detectable on histology, and notation of abnormal appearance of the membranes grossly acts as a reminder to the pathologist at microscopic examination.

Infarcts: In addition to the documenting of gross ledions, in the instance when potential infarcts (Fig. 3.4) are identified central and peripheral lesions should be sampled for histology.

The suspected infarcts should also be qualified, where possible, as to whether they are recent or remote. If a central hemorrhage is detected in the lesion, it should also be described and a sample should be taken for histological examination. When histology confirms that the hemorrhage is encased by infarction, the proposed term infarction hematoma should be used. Infarcts can be suspected by their generally pyramidal shape and usual involvement of the basal parenchyma or maternal floor of the placenta. Gross chronologic dating of infarcts is easier in the fixed placenta because the lesions are better demarcated.

3.1 Microscopic Examination of the Placenta and Fetal Membranes

In our practice, tissue samples are fixed in 10% neutral (pH 7.2) formalin solution and embedded in paraffin. Sections were stained with hematoxylin and eosin. Histological examination of pieces, standardly cut from different parts of the placenta (fetal and maternal surfaces of the placenta in the central and peripheral parts, extraplacental membranes, and umbilical cord) in a light-optical microscope, the maturity of the placenta, the severity of compensatory-adaptive reactions, and involutive-dystrophic changes were assessed. To assess the severity of certain signs, a semiquantitative method was used: the designation in the form (+++) indicates a high severity of the trait, (++)—moderate, (+)—low. A negative result is indicated by a minus sign (−).

In addition, clinical and anamnestic data given in the directions received from maternity hospitals were analyzed.

Histological 4-μm-thick sections were obtained from paraffin blocks for hematoxylin and eosin.

The Warthin-Starry staining method can be used to identify Treponema pallidum and Listeria monocytogenes in histological material [2, 3]. According our experience, PAS method is useful for detection most of the fungi, mycoplasma, and chlamydia [4].

The immunohistochemical staining method was carried out according to the recommendations of the manufacturers contained in the protocols given in the accompanying documents for the reagents and the manual "Immunohistochemical Staining Methods" [5].

References

1. Khong TY, Mooney EE, Ariel I, Balmus NCM, et al. Sampling and definitions of placental lesions. Amsterdam Placental Workshop Group Consensus statement. Arch Pathol Lab Med. 2016;140(7):698–713. https://doi.org/10.5858/arpa.2015-0225-CC.

2. Manual of histologic staining methods of the armed forces institute of pathology. 3rd ed. New York: McGraw-Hill; 1969. p. 238–40.
3. Rosa MF, Quintella LP, Ferreira LC, Cuzzi T. Immunohistochemical detection of Treponema pallidum in skin samples with clinical and histopathological correlations and Warthin-Starry staining critical analysis. An Bras Dermatol. 2023;98(4):480–6. https://doi.org/10.1016/j.abd.2022.02.008.
4. Zinserling VA. Infectious pathology of the respiratory tract. Springer; 2021. p. 13–20.
5. Kumar GL, editor. Immunohistochemical staining methods. Carpinteria: Lars Rudbeck Dako North America, Incorporated; 2009, 162p.

4 Placental Microbiome and Intra-amniotic Infection

The unique placental microbiome resembles the microflora of the oral cavity and consists of non-pathogenic commensal microflora types: Firmicutes, Tenericutes, Proteobacteria, Bacteroides, and Fusobacteria [1]. At the same time, these microorganisms, due to immunosuppression during pregnancy, may be etiological factors of ascending amniotic infection [2, 3]. Bacterial placentitis arising from hematogenous infection can be caused by coagulase-positive staphylococci, streptococci, pneumococci, *Haemophilus influenzae*, *Escherichia*, *Salmonella*, Clostridium perfringens, Corynebacteria, Fusobacteria, Bacteroids, Campylobacter fetus, *Streptobacilli*, *Gardnerella* [4, 5].

In our microbiological study of 115 placentas with placental membranes with standard cultures for aerobic microbiota, the most frequently detected bacteria were: *Escherichia* coli (46 observations—40%), enterococci (32 observations—27%), their combination (22 observations—19%). In six cases (5%), the presence of *Staphylococcus aureus* was noted, and in two cases (2%)—*Streptococcus viridans*.

Intra-amniotic infection (IAI) is an infection resulting in the inflammation of any combination of the amniotic fluid, the placenta, the fetus itself, the fetal membranes, umbilical cord, or the decidua. Inflammatory changes in the placentas and fetal membranes are noted in 96% of cases, with basal deciduitis detected in 54% of cases, acute chorioamnionitis in 46%, and villitis in 17%. In the placenta and fetal membranes of fetuses that died antenatally, the etiology of infection is represented mainly by a combined viral and bacterial flora (52%) [6].

The number of placental macrophages varies according to pregnancy trimesters. In the third trimester, they over-express T cell chemokines (CXCL9, CXCL10, CXCL11) associated with altered villous architecture [7, 8]. Mezouar et al. (2021) found that the balance between TNF and IL-10, as pro- and anti-inflammatory cytokines, respectively, is reoriented toward inflammatory response in chorioamnionitis. The expression of CD163, an M2 marker, on placental macrophages is higher in grade III than in grade II chorioamnionitis. It was also shown that CD14+ placental macrophages from patients with chorioamnionitis are unable to form multinuclear giant cells [9]. This defect is partially corrected by incubating placental macrophages with control trophoblast supernatants, thus demonstrating the role of the placenta microenvironment in multinuclear giant cell formation [10]. Placental macrophages may be also pathogenic through the release of extracellular traps (ET) in group B Streptococcus infection [11]. The release of placenta ET depends on actin polymerization and reactive oxygen species. Placenta ETs contain matrix metalloproteinases which are released during infection and lead to breakdown of extracellular matrix and placenta lesions [12]. This way of

V. Zinserling et al., *Placentitis and Perinatal Infections*,
https://doi.org/10.1007/978-3-031-80553-0_4

response of placenta macrophages to infection is shared with other placenta cells. Indeed, it was reported that the expression of cytonemes, actin-based filopodia that mediate paracrine signaling, by placenta mast cells in response to infection with anti-bacterial properties [9, 12]. The role in infections by intracellular bacteria that present a placenta tropism is less well documented. During Listeria monocytogenes infection, a ubiquitous intracellular gram-positive bacterium responsible of listeriosis macrophages from placenta were found permissive [13, 14]. It has been also provided evidence that during infection due *Brucella* sp. or *C. burnetii*, in placental macrophages pathogen was found [15, 16]. Mezouar et al. (2019) recently showed that CD14+ macrophages from at term healthy placentas infected ex vivo by *C. burnetii* eliminate bacteria within 9 days. This elimination is associated with their polarization in M1 cells and is related to the production of IFN-γ [12]. The microbicidal activity of macrophages from at term placentas may account for the fact that the transmission from mother to fetus mainly occurs during first and second trimesters, not during the third trimester. But to date, the factors that govern the mechanisms of infection, the resistance, and/or the susceptibility to these bacteria in decidual macrophages are still unknown [17].

In the past, an infection of the amnion and chorion or both was dubbed chorioamnionitis. In 2015, a proposal was made by an expert panel that, instead of clinical chorioamnionitis, the name intrauterine inflammation or infection or both be used, abbreviated as Triple I or simply IAI. However, the abbreviation IAI did not gain popularity, and this article uses the term chorioamnionitis. Chorioamnionitis may arise prior to, during, or following labor. It can present as a chronic, subacute, or acute infection. Its clinical presentation is generally referred to as acute chorioamnionitis [18].

According to Khong et al. (2016), the participants recognized that ascending intrauterine infection is clinically important and that its histologic documentation forms a substantial amount of the clinically indicated placental pathology workload. There was agreement to emphasize that histologic chorioamnionitis may not be equivalent to clinical chorioamnionitis. There was, however, debate around whether to describe the stage and grade of inflammation in the reports [19].

Acute chorioamnionitis (Fig. 4.1), the histopathological counterpart of the clinical diagnosis of intraamniotic infection is diagnosed in 50–60% of women with preterm premature rupture of membranes (PPROM) [20–22]. As chorioamnionitis poses a danger to the fetus by promoting early-onset sepsis and neonatal morbidities, such as bacterial pneumonia (Fig. 4.2), cystic periventricular leukomalacia, and cerebral palsy, its early and accurate diagnosis and treatment are indispensable [23]. Moreover, the mother is also at risk of developing sepsis, and may request admission to an intensive care unit [24]. Currently, serial measurements of C-reactive protein and leucocytes serve to monitor the development of infection in women with PPROM.

In 2018, the American Academy of Pediatrics (AAP) revised national guidelines to recommend several approaches to identify infants ≥35 weeks gestational age (GA) at increased risk of early-onset sepsis (EOS). Two of these approaches include: (1) categorical risk factor assessment and (2) multivariate risk assessment [25]. Each approach aims to identify infants with EOS to allow appropriate intervention and treatment while minimizing the identification of uninfected infants to avoid unnecessary antibiotic exposure, laboratory evaluations, and disruption of maternal/infant bonding. However, as of 2017, the American College of Obstetrics and Gynecology

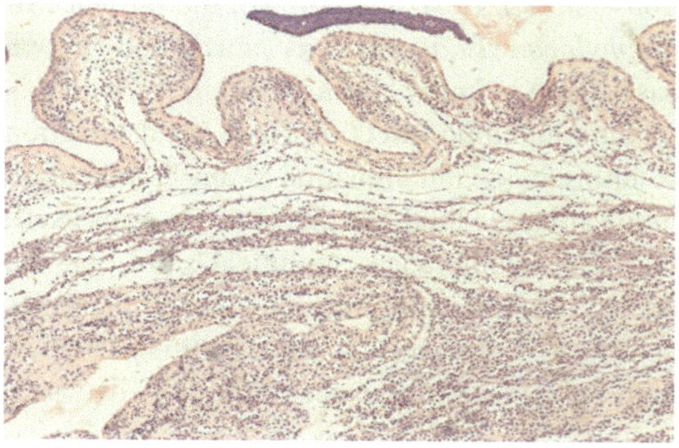

Fig. 4.1 Acute chorioamnionitis, H&E, ×50

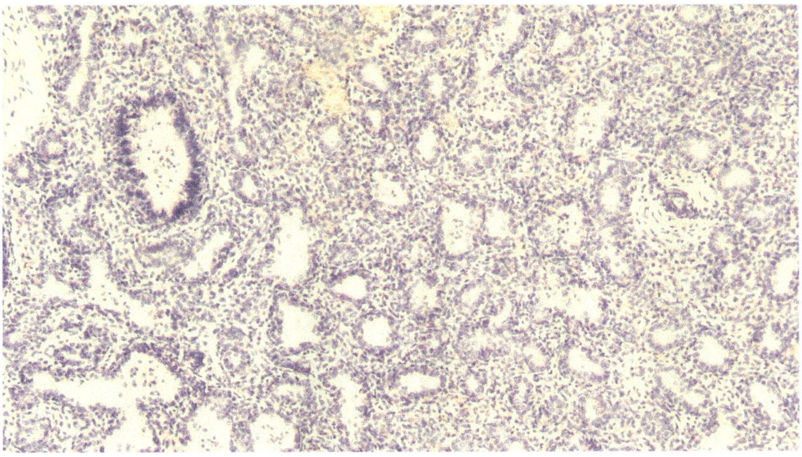

Fig. 4.2 Congenital unspecified pneumonia, antenatal fetal death, 23 weeks of gestation, H&E, ×200

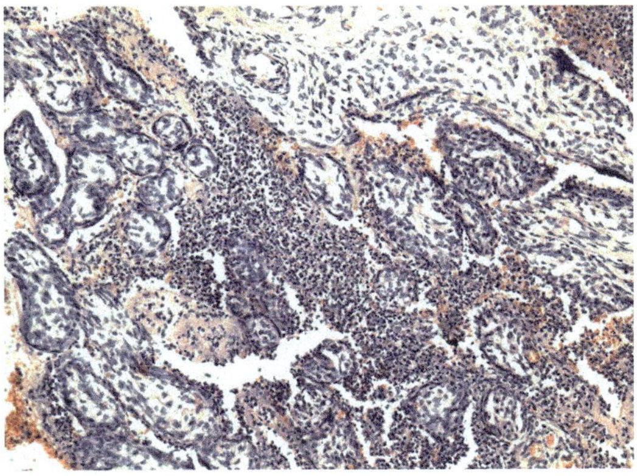

Fig. 4.3 Acute subchorionitis, H&E, ×200

(ACOG) recommends transitioning away from the terminology and historical criteria for clinical chorioamnionitis and instead recommends new clinical criteria (see methods), which are used to diagnosis women with suspected intraamniotic infection [26].

The presence of neutrophils in the subchorial intervillous space or beneath the chorion laeve layer in the absence of inflammation elsewhere is not synonymous with acute chorioamnionitis and should be reported as subchorionitis (Fig. 4.3).

Patchy accumulation of more than occasional polymorphonuclear leukocytes in the subchorionic fibrin and/or at the choriodecidual interface in the decidua represents an early stage of the response to amniotic fluid infection, whereas chorioamnionitis means exactly what it says, that is to say, inflammation in the chorion and amnion.

In our observations maternal signs of an ascending amniotic infection (acute chorioamnionitis, intervillitis) were noted in 80% of cases with non-induced preterm birth 22–27 weeks of gestation (Fig. 4.4, row I), in 62%—with induced preterm birth 22–27 weeks of gestation (Fig. 4.4, row II), in 58%—with preterm birth 28–36 weeks of gestation (Fig. 4.4, row III), and in 51%—with preterm birth 28–36 weeks of gestation by cesarean section sections (Fig. 4.4, row IV). At the same time, in urgent delivery, acute chorioamnionitis was detected in 31% of placentas and fetal membranes (Fig. 4.4, row V) [6].

Infectious processes caused by viruses and other, mainly intracellular, microorganisms (mycoplasmas and/or chlamydia) were detected in non-induced preterm birth 22–27 weeks of gestation in 19%, in induced preterm birth 22–27 weeks of gestation in 37%, in non-induced preterm birth 28–36 weeks of gestation in 41%, in preterm birth 28–36 weeks of gestation by cesarean section in 48%, and 24% for term birth.

In addition to acute chorioamnionitis, it is important to identify funisitis involving umbilical vein, arteria, and stromal funisitis (Fig. 4.5).

To determine the risks of infectious complications for both the woman and the newborn child, the method of detecting neutrophils is used, in particular in the vessels of the umbilical cord. Using *artificial intelligence*, the umbilical cord is identified in scanned slides, then the vessels of the umbilical cord are segmented and neutrophils are detected, followed by an assessment of the severity of inflammation (Fig. 4.6).

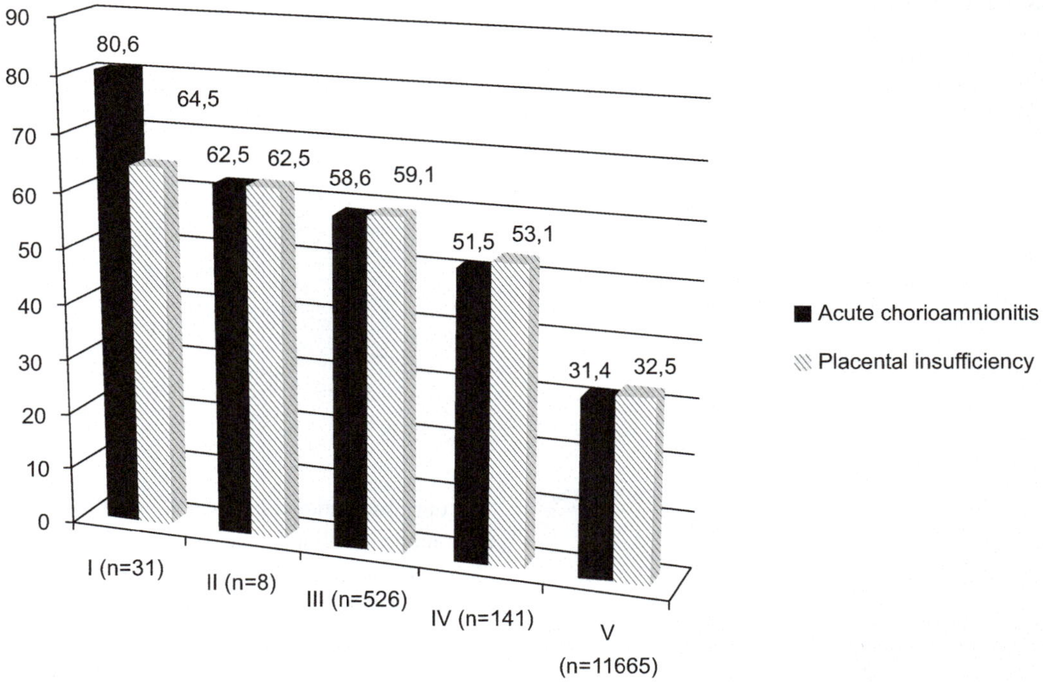

Fig. 4.4 Distribution of ascending amniotic infection and placental insufficiency (%) on morphological material during screening examination of the placenta and extra-placental membranes (row I—non-induced preterm birth 22–27 weeks of gestation; row II—induced preterm birth 22–27 weeks of gestation; row III—non-induced preterm birth 28–36 weeks of gestation; row IV—preterm birth 28–36 weeks of gestation by cesarean section; row V—term birth)

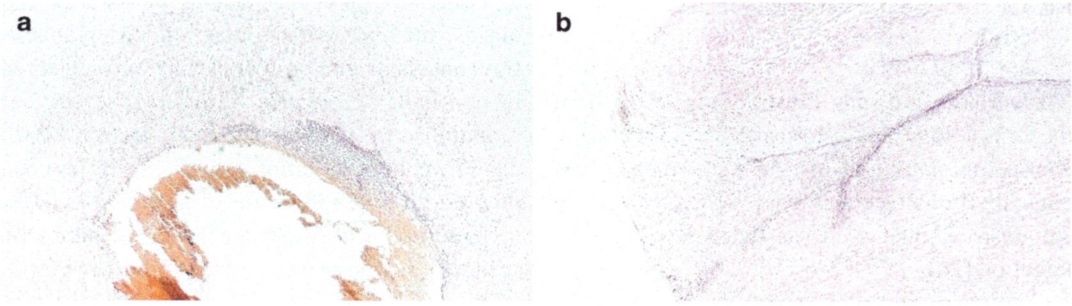

Fig. 4.5 Acute funisitis involving umbilical vein (**a**) and arteria (**b**), H&E, ×50

Artificial intelligence

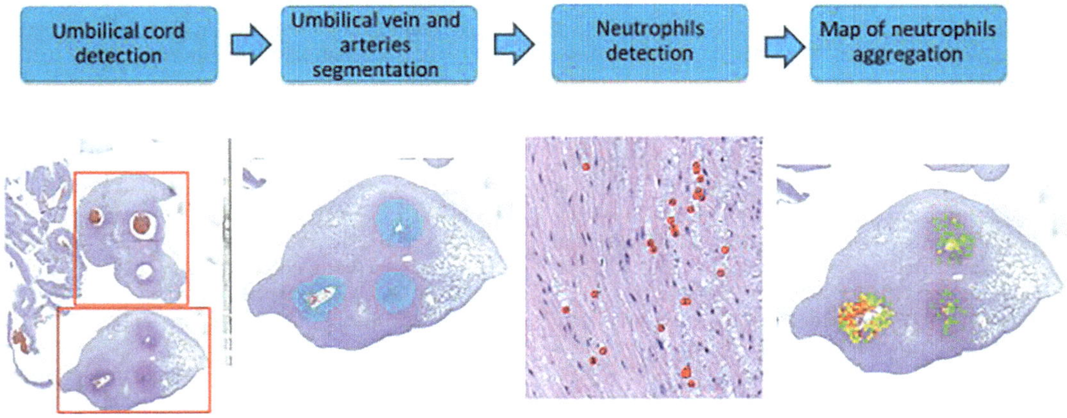

Fig. 4.6 Algorithm of artificial intelligence method for neutrophil detection in H&E slides

References

1. Aagaard K, Ma J, Antony KM, Ganu R, Petrosino J, Versalovic J. The placenta harbors a unique microbiome. Sci Transl Med. 2014;6(237):237ra65. https://doi.org/10.1126/scitranslmed.3008599.
2. Antony KM, Ma J, Mitchell KB, Racusin DA, Versalovic J, Aagaard K. The preterm placental microbiome varies in association with excess maternal gestational weight gain. Am J Obstet Gynecol. 2015;212(5):653.e1–16. https://doi.org/10.1016/j.ajog.2014.12.041.
3. Theis KR, Romero R, Winters AD, Greenberg JM, et al. Does the human placenta delivered at term have a microbiota? Results of cultivation, quantitative real-time PCR, 16S rRNA gene sequencing, and metagenomics. Am J Obstet Gynecol. 2019;220(3):267.e1–267.e39. https://doi.org/10.1016/j.ajog.2018.10.018.
4. Mendz GL, Kaakoush NO, Quinlivan JA. Bacterial aetiological agents of intra-amniotic infections and preterm birth in pregnant women. Front Cell Infect Microbiol. 2013;3:58. https://doi.org/10.3389/fcimb.2013.00058.
5. Verma I, Avasthi K, Berry V. Urogenital infections as a risk factor for preterm labor: a hospital-based case-control study. J Obstet Gynaecol India. 2014;64(4):274–8. https://doi.org/10.1007/s13224-014-0523-6.
6. Kolobov A, Merkulova A, Zinserling V. Intra-amniotic inflammation can influence late abortion and preterm labor. Virchows Arch. 2011;459(Suppl. 1):S124.
7. Kim J-S, Romero R, Kim MR, Kim YM, Friel L, Espinoza J, Kim CJ. Involvement of Hofbauer cells and maternal T cells in villitis of unknown aetiology. Histopathology. 2008;52:457–64. https://doi.org/10.1111/j.1365-2559.2008.02964.x.
8. Förger F, Villiger PM. Immunological adaptations in pregnancy that modulate rheumatoid arthritis disease activity. Nat Rev Rheumatol. 2020;16:113–22. https://doi.org/10.1038/s41584-019-0351-2.
9. Mezouar S, Katsogiannou M, Amara AB, Bretelle F, Mege J-L. Placental macrophages: origin, heterogeneity, function and role in pregnancy-associated infections. Placenta. 2021;103:94–103. https://doi.org/10.1016/j.placenta.2020.10.017.
10. Amara AB, Gorvel L, Baulan K, Derain-Court J, et al. Placental macrophages are impaired in chorioamnionitis, an infectious pathology of the placenta. J Immunol. 2013;191(11):5501–14. https://doi.org/10.4049/jimmunol.1300988.
11. Doster RS, Sutton JA, Rogers LM, Aronoff DM, Gaddy JA. Streptococcus agalactiae induces placental macrophages to release extracellular traps loaded with tissue remodeling enzymes via an oxidative burst-dependent mechanism. mBio. 2018;9(6):e02084–18. https://doi.org/10.1128/mBio.02084-18.
12. Mezouar S, Vitte J, Gorvel L, Amara AB, Desnues B, Mege JL. Mast cell cytonemes as a defense mechanism against Coxiella burnetii. mBio. 2019;10(2):e02669–18. https://doi.org/10.1128/mBio.02669-18.
13. Robbins JR, Skrzypczynska KM, Zeldovich VB, Kapidzic M, Bakardjiev AI. Placental syncytiotrophoblast constitutes a major barrier to vertical transmission of Listeria monocytogenes. PLoS Pathog. 2010;6(1):e1000732. https://doi.org/10.1371/journal.ppat.1000732.
14. Zeldovich VB, Clausen CH, Bradford E, Fletcher DA, Maltepe E, Robbins JR, Bakardjiev AI. Placental syncytium forms a biophysical barrier against pathogen

invasion. PLoS Pathog. 2013;9(12):e1003821. https://doi.org/10.1371/journal.ppat.1003821.
15. Meador VP, Hagemoser WA, Deyoe BL. Histopathologic findings in Brucella abortus-infected, pregnant goats. Am J Vet Res. 1988;49(2):274–80.
16. Osburn BI, Kennedy PC. Pathologic and immunologic responses of the fetal lamb to Brucella ovis. Pathol Vet. 1966;3(2):110–36. https://doi.org/10.1177/030098586600300202.
17. Mezouar S, Benammar I, Boumaza A, Diallo AB, Chartier C, Buffat C, Boudjarane J, Halfon P, Katsogiannou M, Mege J-L. Full-term human placental macrophages eliminate Coxiella burnetii through an IFN-γ autocrine loop. Front Microbiol. 2019;10:2434. https://doi.org/10.3389/fmicb.2019.02434.
18. Lukanović D, Batkoska M, Kavšek G, Druškovič M. Clinical chorioamnionitis: where do we stand now? Front Med (Lausanne). 2023;10:1191254. https://doi.org/10.3389/fmed.2023.1191254.
19. Khong TY, Mooney EE, Ariel I, Balmus NCM, et al. Sampling and definitions of placental lesions. Amsterdam Placental Workshop Group Consensus statement. Arch Pathol Lab Med. 2016;140(7):698–713. https://doi.org/10.5858/arpa.2015-0225-CC.
20. Brun R, Girsberger J, Rothenbühler M, Argyle C, Hutmacher J, Haslinger C, Leeners B. Wearable sensors for prediction of intraamniotic infection in women with preterm premature rupture of membranes: a prospective proof of principle study. Arch Gynecol Obstet. 2023;308(5):1447–56. https://doi.org/10.1007/s00404-022-06753-4.
21. Kim CJ, Romero R, Chaemsaithong P, Chaiyasit N, Yoon BH, Kim YM. Acute chorioamnionitis and funisitis: definition, pathologic features, and clinical significance. Am J Obstet Gynecol. 2015;213(4 Suppl):S29–52. https://doi.org/10.1016/j.ajog.2015.08.040.
22. Kim SA, Park KH, Lee SM. Non-invasive prediction of histologic chorioamnionitis in women with preterm premature rupture of membranes. Yonsei Med J. 2016;57(2):461–8. https://doi.org/10.3349/ymj.2016.57.2.461.
23. Randis TM, Rice MM, Myatt L, Tita ATN, et al. Incidence of early-onset sepsis in infants born to women with clinical chorioamnionitis. J Perinat Med. 2018;46(8):926–33. https://doi.org/10.1515/jpm-2017-0192.
24. Tita AT, Andrews WW. Diagnosis and management of clinical chorioamnionitis. Clin Perinatol. 2010;37(2):339–54. https://doi.org/10.1016/j.clp.2010.02.003.
25. Puopolo KM, Benitz WE, Zaoutis TE. Management of neonates born at ≥35 0/7 weeks' gestation with suspected or proven early-onset bacterial sepsis. Pediatrics. 2018;142(6):e20182894. https://doi.org/10.1542/peds.2018-2894.
26. ACOG. Committee Opinion No. 712 summary: intrapartum management of intraamniotic infection. Obstet Gynecol. 2017;130(2):490–2.

5 Transplacental Transmission Infections: General Consideration. Bacterial Infections

5.1 Transplacental Transmission. General Considerations

The pathogenesis of lesions and substantial consequences resulting from viral infections during pregnancy still remain largely uncharacterized, in particular, relatively little is known about the fundamental biology behind the vertical transmission of viruses. Although it has been widely accepted that the placenta acts as a defensive barrier against viral insults, the molecular mechanisms underlying control of placental infection are still poorly understood. Several hypotheses have been proposed to explain how the placenta avoids viral infections under normal conditions based on human and mouse studies, which include but not limited to the physical or anatomical defenses, intrinsic cellular mechanisms, the constitutive release of antimicrobial immunomodulators, and so on [1]. Moreover, great progress has been achieved regarding the transplacental transmission and pathogenesis of TORCH pathogens, especially those advanced insights obtained in animal models [2–4].

The following ways of antenatal infection of the fetus are considered: transplacental (hematogenous) and contact (through infection of amniotic fluid or at the time of delivery) [5–8].

The possibility of infection of the fetus with a low viral load in the mother is associated with a number of factors—the presence of other infections in the woman, including sexually transmitted infections, poor maternal nutrition, smoking, injecting drug use [5, 9–11]. In addition, inflammatory processes in the placenta play a role (acute chorioamnionitis, villitis) [12].

The factual materials confirm the position on the exceptional practical and theoretical significance of taking into account the functional and structural characteristics of the placenta both in medical and diagnostic work with individual patients and in scientific analysis. At the same time, a number of extremely important questions do not have sufficiently substantiated answers; moreover, these questions, despite their obviousness, are rarely formulated.

Sexually transmitted infections (STI) refer to a variety of clinical syndromes and infections caused by pathogens that can be acquired and transmitted through sexual activity. STIs are common global causes of illness, long-term disability, and death with serious medical and psychological consequences for millions of people [13]. They have far-reaching health, social, and economic consequences in countries and communities where socio-economic conditions are poor [14, 15]. There are over 30 bacterial, viral, and parasitic pathogens that can be transmitted sexually. The global prevalence of bacterial STI among individuals aged 15–49 years is annually estimated by the World Health Organization

Section 5.2.3: Tuberculosis (in collaboration with Y.R. Zyuzya).

V. Zinserling et al., *Placentitis and Perinatal Infections*,
https://doi.org/10.1007/978-3-031-80553-0_5

(WHO) using data from regions with robust case-based surveillance systems and population-based studies. In 2020, the overall world prevalence was 3.2% [2.7–3.9%] for *Chlamydia trachomatis*, 0.7% [0.5–1.1%] for *Neisseria gonorrhoeae*, and 0.6% [0.5–0.7%] for syphilis. The WHO European Region exhibited the lowest STI prevalence among all WHO regions for both genders, with values of 2.7% [2.2–3.5] for *Chlamydia trachomatis*, 0.3% [0.1–0.5] for *Neisseria gonorrhoeae*, and 0.11% [0.09–0.13] for syphilis. Additionally, lymphogranuloma venereum (LGV, CT serovar L1–L3) has been associated with several outbreaks in Europe; the infection, although notifiable, is considerably underreported [16]. In addition, over 500 million people are estimated to have a viral STI such as herpes simplex virus type 2 (HSV-2) or human papillomavirus (HPV) at any point in time [17]. In the developed world, viral infections have become increasingly common and important, whereas bacterial STIs are more common in low- and middle-income countries, but even this is changing with the increasing recognition of viral infections [18].

The high burden of infectious diseases, high infant and maternal mortality, and low-birth weight are among the leading health problems [19–21].

In certain situations, such as influenza, lesions of placenta and fetus occur as result of hematogenic spread of clinically manifest respiratory infection. In other cases without distinct disease of mother pathogenesis of perinatal lesions not always can be clarified.

5.2 Bacterial Infections

5.2.1 Syphilis

Syphilis is among the most common STI worldwide and is also one of the leading preventable and treatable causes of infant morbidity and mortality. First descriptions of inborn syphilis appeared centuries ago with numerous descriptions of histopathological changes both in placentas and newborns/fetuses although we have to note the lack of confirmation in old studies that all descriptions of lesions were due to *Treponema pallidum*.

The maternal and congenital syphilis might contribute to the adverse maternal and child health profiles of indigenous populations in several world regions.

Confirmed congenital syphilis is defined as a case that is laboratory confirmed with one of the following:

1. Non-treponemal test results in neonates ≥ fourfold compared to mothers.
2. Direct identification of *T. pallidum* by specimen from the placenta, umbilical cord, secretions or lesions from infants using darkfield or fluorescent antibody test.
3. Pathologic findings from placenta or umbilical cord consistent with congenital syphilis [22].

Congenital syphilis, which is transmitted from mother to child during pregnancy, can lead to several adverse fetal outcomes, such as stillbirths, neonatal deaths, preterm births, low-birth weight, and congenital infection in infants. The World Health Organization (WHO) has been achieving encouraging results in response to the global initiative to eliminate vertical transmission of syphilis [23]. However, the burden of maternal and congenital syphilis remains substantial and heterogeneous between WHO Regions, countries, and specific population groups [21, 24].

Updated estimates of the burden of maternal and congenital syphilis showed a stable global prevalence of maternal syphilis and a slight decrease in the rate of congenital syphilis (although still high) between 2012 and 2016. These occurred in parallel with an increase in the coverage of antenatal care, screening for syphilis during pregnancy, and treatment of maternal syphilis, although regional disparities persisted [24]. In 2016, for example, while the prevalence of maternal syphilis was 0.10% in Europe, it was 0.86% in the Americas and 1.52% in Africa. Rates of congenital syphilis reached 19, 339, and 1119 per 100,000 live births, in Europe, the Americas, and Africa, respectively [24].

The Russell et al. [25] found 62 studies in 12 countries, but only six reported data on maternal and congenital syphilis; four described the prevalence of maternal syphilis through cross-sectional surveys. Data on congenital syphilis were even more limited and restricted to two publications: a Brazilian government report of 17 cases of congenital syphilis among Indigenous Peoples, notified between 2000 and 2005, and a feasibility study for rapid testing of syphilis in remote areas of the Brazilian Amazon, which detected two congenital syphilis and 19 maternal syphilis cases, suggesting limited access to antenatal care, and underreporting of cases. Both the assessed reviews reinforce the global invisibility of maternal and congenital syphilis in indigenous peoples. The scarcity of studies on this topic remains an obstacle to estimating ethnic–racial inequalities in the disease burden, identifying its determinants, and defining priority groups for social and health public policy implementation [25].

On macroscopic examination, the placenta is usually hyperplastic, thickened, and on section, the placental tissue is pale and light yellow. Histological examination of the placenta can be of great help, since the histopathological triad, including: (1) enlarged, cell-rich villi, (2) proliferative changes in the fetal vessels, (3) acute or chronic villitis, can be interpreted as a characteristic manifestation of syphilitic infection in the placenta (Fig. 5.1) [26].

Greco et al. [27] showed increased histiocytes and Hofbauer cells in addition to a few plasmocytes and lymphocytes, necrosis, and agglutination of villi with intervillous fibrin and granulocytes. All cases of syphilis showed variable degrees of villous fibrosis and sclerosis and obliteration of blood vessels.

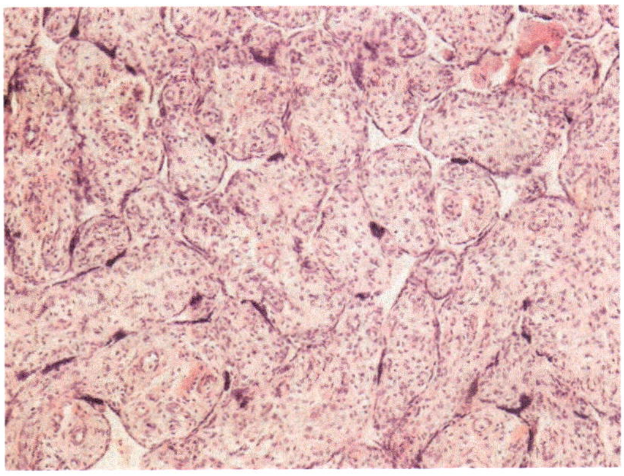

Fig. 5.1 Syphilitic placentitis, fibrosis and proliferative inflammation H&E, ×100

In addition, a number of authors note that in some cases, the placenta with intrauterine syphilitic infection of the fetus may not be generally changed, but there is a violation of the maturation of the villi. In this condition, either groups of immature villi are detected or their accelerated development with excessive vascularization and even angiomatosis.

Among first-trimester abortions in spontaneous miscarriages in women with positive RPR/FTA-ABS tests, 100% of placentas had plasmacytic deciduitis, 33% had an incomplete histopathological triad (enlarged, cell-rich villi, focal acute villitis). Silver and PCR diagnostics were negative in all abortuses. Among the placentas of the fetuses of the second and third trimesters of pregnancy in women with positive RPR/FTA-ABS tests, 11% of the afterbirths showed a complete histopathological triad, 14%—an incomplete (two signs), and 74% were histologically negative. Plasmacytic deciduitis occurred in 14% and acute chorioamnionitis in 31%. In 50% with a complete histopathological triad, a spirochete was identified using silvering. These were either single microorganisms or small groups of treponemas with predominant localization in the fibrous stroma of the villi with acute villitis or intervillitis. Treponemal DNA in placentas with a complete histopathological triad was identified by PCR in 100% [28].

In placentas with an incomplete histopathological triad, all attempts to detect treponema by silvering were unsuccessful, but in 20% treponemal DNA was identified by PCR. PCR-positive placentas had enlarged, cell-rich villi and proliferative changes in fetal vessels without villitis [28].

Among placentas of the second and third trimesters of pregnancy without a histopathological triad, silver staining did not reveal treponema. PCR revealed treponemal DNA in 4% of cases in placentas with acute chorioamnionitis and proliferative changes in fetal vessels. In the absence of a histopathological triad, these changes were regarded as non-specific after fetal death [28].

Necrotizing funisitis, which is associated with increased rates of stillbirth, perinatal infection, and preterm delivery, is sometimes accompanied with congenital syphilis. Macroscopically, layer-by-layer dissection reveals rings and yellow-white stripes parallel to the vessels of the funiculus. Inflammation of the umbilical cord is characterized by the release of inflammatory cells from the intima into the Warton's jelly with neutrophil degeneration, basophilic debris, and sometimes extensive calcification that forms semicircles or rings around one or more umbilical vessels. Immunohistochemistry (IHC) has been used to detect *Treponema pallidum* in the placenta and umbilical cord [29]. Benirschke et al. [26] showed that in his material necrotizing funisitis is common and in some cases there was indeed a combination with congenital syphilis, but in other cases, despite an exhaustive examination, including VDRL, etiological agents were not identified. In a study conducted by Qureshi et al. [28], these data are confirmed by the fact that only one of the 45 cases of necrotizing funiculitis in a woman was diagnosed with syphilis [28].

Guarner et al. [30] reported that 11% of neonates born from maternal syphilis had necrotizing funisitis with *T. pallidum* [30]. Their conclusion is supported by data that the development of necrotic funiculitis in 62% is preceded by premature rupture of the membranes and in 100% necrotizing funiculitis is combined with acute chorioamnionitis.

Based on the literature data, it can be concluded that the verification of fetal and newborn syphilis is quite difficult. There is no data on changes of clinical course and pathological picture in fetal and placental syphilis during last decades. The placenta is sometimes examined after a clinical diagnosis of early congenital syphilis has been made, while it is necessary to develop criteria for detecting syphilitic lesions of the placenta and fetal organs under conditions of screening and morphological verification in case of autolytic changes.

Epidemiological and social aspects play a large role in realizing the risk of developing congenital syphilis and are closely related to medical prerequisites. Long-term observations of most researchers show that the prognosis for a child depends on the stage of the disease in the mother and the gestational age at which syphilis was detected, as well as the start date and treatment tactics. If the mother has untreated syphilis with a prescription of 2 years or more, in 50% of cases live births, children are born without signs of infection. If a pregnant woman has untreated primary or secondary syphilis, this can lead to 50% stillbirth or death of the child in the neonatal period. At the same time, at an early stage of untreated tertiary syphilis, healthy newborns are born in 20–40% of cases, 40% of children have congenital syphilis, 20% are born prematurely, and 16% are stillbirths and death of children in the first 4 weeks of life. In late stage tertiary syphilis, only 10% of children have congenital syphilis, 10% are stillbirths, and in 1% neonatal deaths are noted [31].

Tendencies and features of the increase in antibody titer in women who gave birth to children with congenital syphilis were revealed. It was also noted that in patients with primary infection, a reversion of the level of antibodies in serum is more often observed than in patients with reinfection. Any woman who tests positive for antibodies 1–2 years after treatment for primary or secondary syphilis should be retreated. Reversion depends on the serum antibody titer before treatment and on the stage of the disease.

Drug dependence can give a false positive result in non-specific biological tests for syphilis, which complicates the interpretation of the adequacy of therapy in patients with a history of syphilis and continuing to take drugs.

Serological IgM tests are unsatisfactory for identifying reinfection, as IgM-specific antibodies may remain positive for up to 2 years after treatment, and reinfection is associated with a reduced IgM response. At the same time, a normal level of IgM antibodies in a newborn does not exclude the presence of a congenital infection [31].

5.2.1.1 Fetal Syphilis and Congenital Syphilis: Clinical Manifestations and Morphological Changes

Great difficulties arise if it is necessary to confirm syphilis in an autopsy material, which is obtained after intrauterine death of the fetus more than 24 h before delivery. The most likely in these cases is the detection of spirochetes by silvering in the liver tissue of the fetus, in rare cases—in the placenta and umbilical cord. It should be noted that in the case of penicillin therapy, pale treponema disappears from the tissues after 10–24 h [32].

Classical signs that allow suspecting congenital syphilis in a fetus that died antenatally include: fetal edema with intrauterine growth retardation (more often with growth retardation), hepatosplenomegaly, microscopically detected perivascular plasmacytic infiltrates and fibrous changes in the subcutaneous vessels, placental hyperplasia [33]. Plasma cell infiltrates are found in soft tissues and in the walls of elastic-type blood vessels. For granulation tissue in this infectious process, the presence of blood vessels and miliary gums is characteristic.

The frequency of birth of premature babies with early congenital syphilis, according to different authors, varies widely: from 6 to 60%, depending on the duration of infection, the duration of the process and the place of study. Preterm infants accounted for 54% of all newborns with early congenital syphilis. Fetal hypotrophy occurs in 28% of patients born to mothers who did not receive antisyphilitic treatment during pregnancy, and in 16% of patients whose mothers received antisyphilitic treatment.

Non-immune fetal edema plays an important role in perinatal pathology, accounting for more than 3% of all causes of perinatal death. The genesis of non-immune edema may be associated with syphilitic infection [33].

Syphilitic pemphigus (pemphigoid)—the only symptom of congenital syphilis with which children are born or which manifests itself in the first days of life, occurs with a frequency of 2–31% children with early congenital syphilis. Bubbles with serous-purulent, and sometimes bloody, contents are localized on the palms and feet, less often on other parts of the skin. At the base of the blisters, there is an infiltrate, so the blisters are surrounded by a reddish-purple rim. After opening the blisters, erosions form in their place, along the periphery of which the fringe of the exfoliated stratum corneum is visible [32].

Diffuse skin infiltration appears in 23% of cases of early congenital syphilis and is localized, except for the palms and feet, on the face (often around the mouth), scalp, buttocks, thighs, elbows, and knees. It is preceded by diffuse erythema of the affected areas.

Syphilitic rhinitis is accompanied by mucosal hyperplasia and its diffuse infiltration by round cell elements and neutrophils, followed by deep ulcerations and damage to the cartilage and bones of the nose. At present, only the dry and catarrhal stages of syphilitic rhinitis are observed, and the ulcerative stage does not occur.

Wegner's osteochondritis, often with lesions of tubular bones, is detected in 2/3 of patients in the first 3 months of life, and after 4 months—only in 5%, periostitis—in every tenth patient with early congenital syphilis.

According to the severity of osteochondritis, there are three stages:

1. a sinuous uneven strip of gray-yellow color 1–2 mm wide;
2. the width of the lesion is up to 5 mm;
3. Parro's pseudoparalysis (separation of the diaphysis from the epiphysis).

In preterm infants, osteochondritis II–III stage predominates.

Clutton was the first to describe symmetrical serous synovitis in congenital syphilis; Verneuil—bursitis; and Charcot—destructive arthritis. With combined intrauterine infection, or the addition of hospital microflora, the formation of purulent foci in the bone tissue is possible [32].

In the gastrointestinal tract, the formation of multiple stenoses due to fibrosis on the background of syphilitic arteritis with perivascular round cell infiltrates in the submucosal and mucous layers, sometimes with ulcerations, is possible. The stomach, small intestine, and colon are most often involved.

Hepatosplenomegaly accompanies syphilitic lesions in 17–29%. Macroscopically, the liver is yellow-brown or whitish-brown in color ("flint liver") of a dense consistency. Histological changes are divided into three types [32].

At the first, cellular infiltration of the capsule and periportal connective tissue, walls of the hepatic veins and bile ducts is determined. The infiltrate consists of histiocytes, plasmocytes, lymphocytes, eosinophils. There is a slight proliferation of stellate reticuloendotheliocytes. Silver staining (Warthin-Starry) shows spirochaetes in portal tracts (Fig. 5.2).

The second type of changes include thickening and infiltration of the liver capsule, proliferation of connective tissue in the lobules, and expansion of the portal tracts. The infiltrative process is concentrated around the bile ducts, where rings of growing connective tissue are formed (syphilitic pericholangitis), and branches of the portal vein (syphilitic periphlebitis). The infiltrates are composed of lymphocytes, plasma cells, histiocytes, and eosinophils. In rare cases, the liver with this type of changes can be reduced in size, have a dense texture and a fine-grained surface.

The third type of changes includes cases with the presence of miliary gums, macroscopically determined in the form of grayish dots (5% of sectional material). Microscopically, foci of necrosis and diffuse inflammatory round cell infiltrates are found in the growing connective tissue.

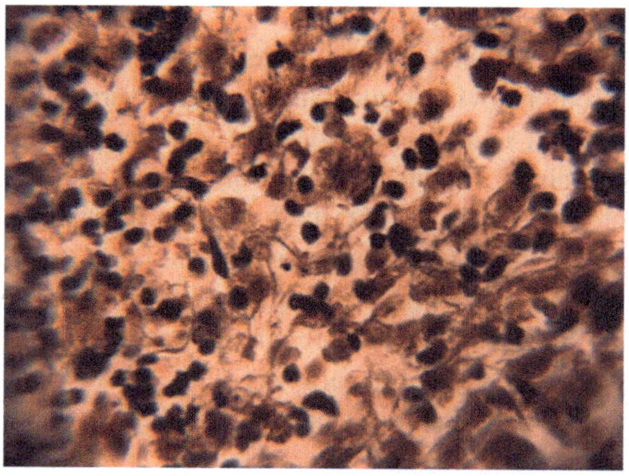

Fig. 5.2 *Treponema pallidum (brown rods)* in liver, silver stain by Warthin-Starry, ×1000

The spleen is dense, its mass increases by ten times or more. Fibrinous deposits on the capsule are often determined (syphilitic perisplenitis), sometimes with hyalinosis of the capsule. Intrafollicular arteries and other vessels are thickened due to productive endarteritis up to obliteration of the lumen.

In the thymus, there is a proliferation of interlobular connective tissue infiltrated with lymphocytes, histiocytes, and plasmocytes. The lobules are small due to the reduced number of lymphocytes in both layers. Hassall's bodies are layered, located both in the cortical and medulla layers.

Infrequently, fibrous (white) pneumonia occurs, which is manifested by thickening of the interalveolar septa, peribronchial, and perivascular tissue with infiltration by lymphocytes, plasma cells, and epithelioid cells. In the lumen of the alveoli, exudate is detected, consisting of neutrophils and alveolar macrophages.

Kidney development is delayed. Glomeruli and tubules are not developed. Specific lesions are described in the form of focal or diffuse interstitial nephritis with round cell infiltration mainly in the cortex, less often in the medulla along the vessels.

Heart damage is manifested by myocarditis with cellular, predominantly plasmacytic, perivascular infiltration, swelling of cells around the vessels.

Among the endocrine glands, the adrenal glands are most commonly involved, with fibrosis of the capsule, fetal cortex, and zona fasciculata of the definitive cortex, while the zona glomeruli is destroyed.

The lesion of the pancreas is characterized by the growth of connective tissue that penetrates between the acini, ducts and islets (interstitial fibrosis). The pattern of the gland can be completely erased, and the consistency can sometimes reach cartilaginous density (Fig. 5.3).

In the central nervous system, productive chronic leptomeningitis, meningoencephalitis, ependymitis are detected. Sometimes, brain tumors develop. There is also progressive hydrocephalus.

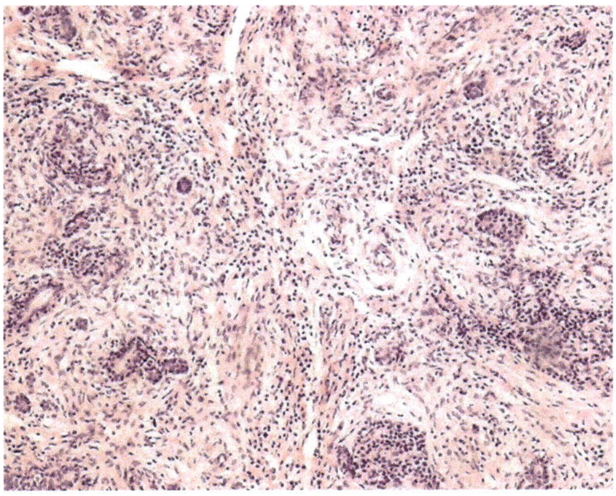

Fig. 5.3 Fibrosis of pancreas with syphilis, H-E, ×100

Eye lesions manifest as chorioretinitis ("salt and pepper" around the periphery of the fundus), uveitis, glaucoma, and optic nerve atrophy.

A congenital syphilis prevention cascade could help visualize the essential services required to prevent congenital syphilis among pregnant women and could help identify opportunities for improvement along the prevention pathway. In addition, a congenital syphilis prevention cascade could also help quantify programmatic successes by describing the number of potential congenital syphilis cases averted each year.

5.2.2 Listeriosis

Listeria monocytogenes is a small Gram-positive bacterium that is transmitted through contaminated food. In pregnancy, it manifests as septicemia, neurolisteriosis, and maternal-fetal infection and may cause maternal fever, premature delivery, fetal loss, and neonatal systemic and central nervous system infections. In a recent outbreak in South Africa, the mortality rate for infants was 28% and for pregnant women it was 8%. Pregnancy-associated morbidity during this outbreak was responsible for 50% of cases presenting to health care [34]. Despite the immaturity of the fetal immune system in early pregnancy, treatment of *L. monocytogenes* in the first trimester after exposure has been shown to improve fetal outcomes [35–37]. By contrast, treatment after the first trimester has not been definitively shown to change the course of the disease for the fetus but is recommended to improve maternal outcomes [38]. This is likely due to enhanced susceptibility of the fetus to *L. monocytogenes* infection after the first trimester and suggests that there are gestational age-specific differences in vertical transmission [39].

After entry through the enteric mucosa, *L. monocytogenes* spreads cell to cell by manipulating actin polymerization. The mechanism of transplacental transmission of the bacterium remains unknown. In ex vivo cultures, the syncytiotrophoblast is highly resistant to infection [40, 41]. The bacterial virulence factors required for entry into other cells (for example, listeriolysin O and internalin B) are not required for entry into human choriocarcinoma trophoblast cell lines [42]. The bacterial internalin protein InlA is important for binding to E-cadherin on primary trophoblasts, but its role in crossing the placental barrier in vivo remains unclear, with differential effects in different animal models [43–45]. Together, these data suggest that transmission across the placental barrier may require additional, yet uncharacterized, bacterial virulence factors. After placental colonization, the bacterium spreads to fetal tissues and can be reseeded back to maternal organs [46]. The secreted bacterial colonization factor internalin P is important for distorting cells and allowing the bacteria to traverse the basement membrane, but the mechanisms of transport across the syncytiotrophoblast to the basement membrane have yet to be characterized [47]. Importantly, fetal infection is associated with placental abscess development and innate immune cell recruitment to the maternal–fetal interface [48].

Macrophages have been shown to spread *L. monocytogenes* infection to other cell types, including endothelial cells, and *L. monocytogenes* cell-to-cell spread is required for infection of the placental/fetal unit [45, 46, 49–53]. Based on their presence at the placental/fetal interface, their phagocytic ability, and their motility, Hofbauer cells are the best candidates for fetal transmission of *L. monocytogenes*. In support of this, Azari et al. [49] found that Hofbauer cells transfer *L. monocytogenes* cells to other primary placental cells, including fetal endothelial cells. *L. monocytogenes*-infected Hofbauer cells upregulate numerous transcripts for chemokines that attract neutrophils, monocytes/macrophages, and T cells, which was confirmed at the protein level with IL-8 [49]. Villitis can lead to infiltration of maternal leukocytes, as evidenced by trafficking of CD8+ cytotoxic T cells in villitis of unknown etiology (VUE) [54, 55]. VUE is also accompanied by increased levels of CXCL9, -10, and -11 (CXCR3 ligands) in HBCs and can lead to fetal death and other complications [56]. There is also an induction of gene expression for these chemokines in *L. monocytogenes*-infected Hofbauer cells. Therefore, it is likely that if infection of chorionic villi is not resolved, exacerbation of inflammation by Hofbauer cells and infiltration of maternal leukocytes may contribute to poor outcomes, such as abortion and preterm birth, observed in listeriosis cases in pregnancy [57].

Macroscopically, the placenta is sometimes enlarged in size and small whitish-yellowish foci scattered throughout the organ are visible; the extraplacental membranes acquire a dirty green color. Microabscesses with areas of necrosis in the center and a palisade-shaped arrangement of histiocytes have been described. Damage to the villi is accompanied by necrosis and thrombosis of the intervillous spaces. Several variants of placental damage in listeriosis are possible: disseminated intervillous placentitis, septic apostematous placentitis, and ascending choriamnionitis (Fig. 5.4) [31].

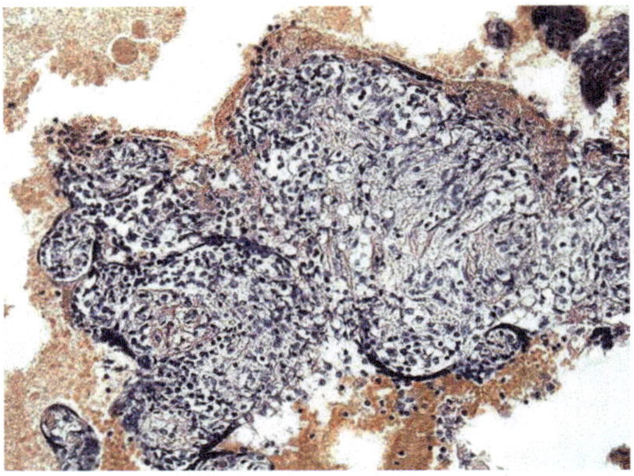

Fig. 5.4 Granuloma in listeriosis in stem villus of placenta. H.-E. ×400

While maternal illness due to listeriosis may be mild, neonatal illness is often severe and may be fatal. Neonatal listeriosis may occur by vertical transmission of *L. monocytogenes* from mother to fetus, either by inhalation of infected amniotic fluid, transplacentally from the maternal circulation or by ascending colonization from the vagina [58, 59]. Though vaginal colonization is rare, nearly half of asymptomatic mothers of infants born with neonatal listeriosis will have a positive vaginal culture for *L. monocytogenes* [60]. This observation is consistent with other perinatal infections like group B Streptococcus (GBS). Similar to GBS, *L. monocytogenes* is likely to result from spread to the vagina from the lower gastrointestinal tract [61–63]. Furthermore, ascending vaginal colonization is supported by the finding of listeria colonization solely in the firstborn of a set of twins [64]. However, hematogenous spread may be more likely, and documented maternal bacteriuria and in utero fetal infection with positive amniotic fluid cultures prior to labor have been recorded [65]. In addition, nosocomial cross-infection has been reported [66–70].

Neonatal listeriosis occurs in approximately 8.6/100,000 of live births and is one of the most common causes of neonatal meningitis [71]. The clinical manifestations of neonatal listeriosis are similar to GBS, and there is a high mortality rate (20–60%) [38, 72–75]. One study reported that 68% of newborns whose mothers were diagnosed with listeriosis as a result of positive cultures from placenta, maternal blood or cervix developed neonatal infection; of those 68.2% made a complete recovery, 12.7% developed long-term neurological sequelae, and the infant mortality rate was 24.5% [38]. Like GBS, there are two forms of the disease in the neonate, early- and late-onset, suggesting different modes of transmission (vertical and nosocomial) [76].

5.2.2.1 Early Onset

Symptoms of early-onset listeriosis occur at a mean of 36 h after birth. In 50–74% of cases, the mother is likely to have had a flu-like illness with symptoms of fever, headache, and myalgia, and isolation of *L. monocytogenes* from maternal blood or genital tract is common (44–89%) ([64, 73, 74]). Neonates with early-onset infection are more frequently born preterm and associated with chorioamnionitis. The fetus presents with clinical features like septicaemia (81–88%), respiratory distress or pneumonia (38%), meningitis (24%), and occasionally disseminated inflammatory granulomatosis (granulomatosis infantisepticum), from which pure culture of *L. monocytogenes* can be obtained ([73, 74, 77]). Granulomatosis infantisepticum was reported for the first time in 1893 (at which time, the disease was named pseudotuberculosis) and is a pathognomonic feature of listeriosis [78, 79].

5.2.2.2 Late Onset

In contrast, late-onset neonatal listeriosis (commonly due to serotype 4b), tends to occur between 5 days and 2 or more weeks postpartum, typically in term neonates [72, 74, 80]. Also typical of these cases is that the neonate is born to asymptomatic mothers with failure to isolate *L. monocytogenes* from maternal cultures [73, 74]. The clinical features may be non-specific, but septicaemia (17–95%) and meningitis (67–93%) are common [68, 81]. Neonatal listeriosis is one of the few congenital infections in which antibiotic therapy can improve outcome [38, 82–84].

The most typical for listeriosis are small foci of inflammation, in the center of which, among the disintegrating leukocytes, a large number of phagocytosed Listeria are detected. Subsequently, the number of leukocytes increases, and an admixture of fibrin is detected in the peripheral areas of such a lesion. At later stages of the process, small growths of granulation tissue appear on the periphery of the lesion, consisting mainly of histiocytes. In the future, this tissue can completely replace the area of necrosis. Listeria is practically not detected in granulation tissue. Macroscopically, listeriomas have the character of small (miliary) yellowish or grayish lesions, sometimes, especially in the liver (merging with each other. Quite often they have a red border. Listeriomas are most easily identified in the liver (Fig. 5.5). Foci of a similar structure can occur in many other organs (Fig. 5.6), then the process is usually called granulomatous sepsis. Along with the granulomatous process, purulent inflammation is sometimes described. Perhaps in this case, secondary pyogenic microflora is involved [32].

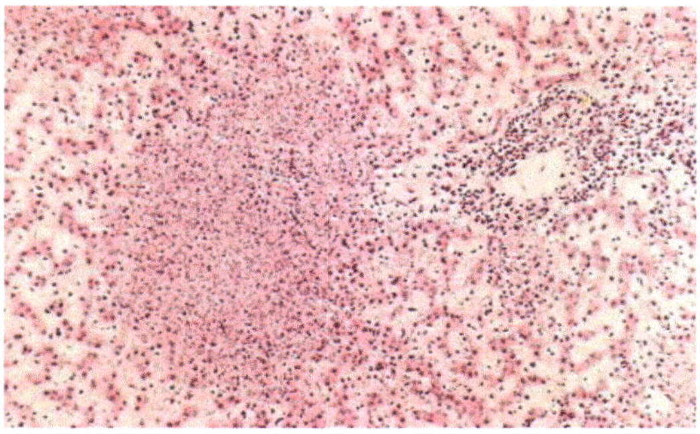

Fig. 5.5 Listeriosis granuloma in liver, H-E, ×200

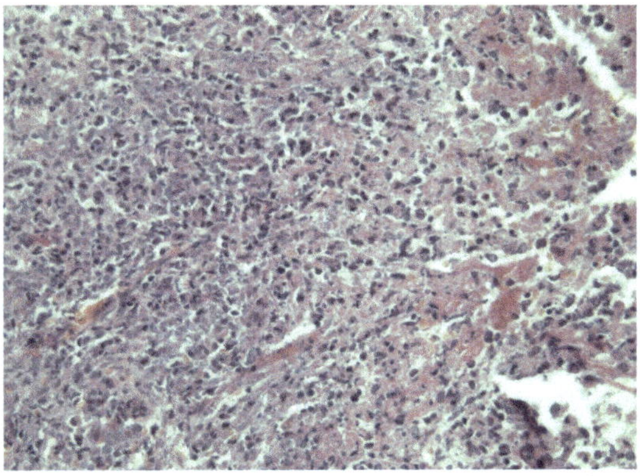

Fig. 5.6 Gut, Granuloma due to *L. monocytogenes*, H-E, ×400

5.2.3 Tuberculosis

Tuberculosis (TB) is the leading infectious cause of mortality globally [85]. The global burden of active TB disease and latent TB infection among pregnant women is not well-known. For 2011, global estimates reported 216,500 pregnant women diagnosed with active TB disease, with the greatest burdens being in World Health Organization African and Southeast-Asian regions [86]. Risk factors for TB infection in pregnant women are the same as risk factors among the general population and include recent exposure to active TB disease, being from a high-burden TB country, and living or working in a high-risk setting. Risk factors for progression from latent TB infection to active TB disease are also the same regardless of pregnancy status: human immunodeficiency virus (HIV) infection, TB infection acquired within the past 2 years, intravenous drug use, and being immunocompromised [87].

Although the incidence of active TB disease is lower in USA and Europe than many other countries, active TB disease during pregnancy remains associated with a substantially elevated risk for poor maternal and fetal outcomes, including a threefold increase in maternal morbidity (e.g., antenatal admission, anemia, and cesarean birth), ninefold increase in miscarriage, twofold increase in preterm birth and low-birth weight, and sixfold increase in perinatal death [86, 88].

The risk of untreated active TB disease on the pregnant woman and on the fetus is greater than the risks of treatment [87]. Congenital TB may be transmitted from a mother with active TB disease to the fetus transplacentally through the bloodstream or lymphatics; it is also possible for M. tuberculosis to be aspirated or ingested through the amniotic fluid during birth. Although rare, congenital TB has a high mortality rate. In one study of 29 cases of perinatal tuberculosis, infant mortality was 38%. Congenital TB may present in the early neonatal period with sepsis or in the first 3 months of life with bronchopneumonia and hepatosplenomegaly. In a separate study, of 32 infants born to 38 mothers with MDR tuberculosis, only 1 infant died of pneumonia. If congenital TB is suspected, evaluation should include histologic and mycobacterial culture of the placenta, in addition to the neonatal evaluation. It is difficult to distinguish between TB acquired as a fetus and TB acquired in the neonatal period.

With hematogenous infection, which can be observed with miliary TB in the mother, the pathogen enters the placenta from the mother's blood through the spiral arteries of the decidual membrane of the placenta or through the endometrial vessels in decidua basalis. This type of infection of the placenta or membranes in most cases is formed antenatally. Prolonged massive bacteremia in the mother contributes to damage to the afterbirth and fetus. In the hematogenic pathway of infection, various structures of the placenta are involved in the pathological process: (1) intervillous space, without predominant localization under the chorial plate; (2) villi and their vessels (villusitis/villitis, vasculitis); (3) the basal plate of the placenta; (4) the true falling shell. With hematogenous infection, the most blood-supplied organs of the fetus that do not border on the external environment are affected—primarily the liver, adrenal glands, kidneys, etc.

The downward path of infection is very rare. The infection penetrates into the tissues of the afterbirth and fetus through the fallopian tube from an inflammatory focus in the abdominal cavity. That is, it can be assumed that with various forms of tuberculous peritonitis, such a path of infection is possible. If the opening of the fallopian tube is covered by the placenta, then the inflammatory process may develop in the basal lamina (including in its vessels), the interstitial space, in villi with damage to fetal tissues. In cases of covering the lumen of the fallopian tube with fetal membranes, initially inflammatory changes may begin in this area of the fetal membranes, then the amniotic fluid becomes infected and further microorganisms spread as in the ascending path.

In addition, a mixed infection pathway is possible.

Placenta with TB, macroscopically, either large foci of cheesy necrosis or multiple miliary lesions is detected on the surfaces of the placenta, in the villous chorion and membranes. As a rule, infection of the placenta occurs hematogenously, less often—from the source of infection in the endometrium. Histological examination in different parts of the organ reveals either small or larger foci of cheesy necrosis, surrounded by a non-specific cellular reaction. In the intervillous space, accumulations of polymorphic cells and fibrin are detected, which in some places undergo cheesy necrosis. In the villi adjacent to such areas, a diffuse proliferation of specific granulation tissue and tuberculous tubercles occur. Often, blood clots form in the vessels of the villi or obliteration of the lumen occurs. When infection spreads from foci in the endometrium, similar changes can be detected in the membranes of the placenta.

Morphological changes in placental TB were described as early as the nineteenth century. In a pregnant woman suffering from TB, the frequency of placental damage directly depends on its course, form and activity of the process. More often (up to 50%) placental lesion is noted in miliary TB, which requires special attention to women with HIV-associated tuberculosis, which is most characterized by acute general miliary TB. In most cases, the basal lamina is involved in the process, including the areas penetrating the interstitial space. Initially, the vascular endothelium of the basal lamina is affected, which is accompanied by the formation of hyaline thrombi. Both productive and exudative-necrotic components may prevail in the foci. The most characteristic is the intravillous localization of foci, and the manifestation of the lesion is thrombosis of chorionic villi vessels. Initially, the destruction of the epithelium of the villi occurs, which undergoes necrotic changes, and then the stroma is affected a second time with the formation of granulomas, tuberculous tubercles, and necrosis sites. Tuberculous lesions of the afterbirth are characterized by a rare umbilical cord lesion, necrotic changes in the walls of blood vessels are described, including the formation of typical tuberculous tubercles with giant multinucleated cells.

As with tuberculous lesions of various organs, with tuberculous lesions of the afterbirth, the so-called specific and non-specific changes are also distinguished. The manifestations of TB of a "specific" nature include granulomas, necrosis, acid-resistant bacteria detected in sections during histobacterioscopic examination. Given the current possibility of using an IHC method using tuberculosis antibodies, the detection of pathogens of the genus mycobacteria in sections of the placenta or afterbirth can also be attributed to this group of manifestations. "Non-specific" changes are manifested by thrombosis of the interstitial space, hemorrhages in the basal membrane, proliferation of chorionic villous stroma cells, fibrosis of their stroma, inflammatory changes of an acute, subacute or productive nature (without elements of granulomatous inflammation), for example, lymphoid, lymphoid-macrophage, lymphoid-leukocyte infiltration). It is noted that "non-specific" changes occur twice as often as "specific" ones.

The identified "specific" morphological changes of the afterbirth, characteristic of tuberculosis lesions, including in cases with bacteriological confirmation of the etiology of the process, species identification of Mycobacterium tuberculosis in the afterbirth material, do not lead mandatory to fetal damage. There are many cases of the birth of a healthy child with confirmed tuberculous inflammation of the afterbirth.

In our opinion, it can be assumed that TB of the afterbirth is probably more common than it is reported in the literature, since huge volume of histological examination of thousands of sections cannot be carried out in each case, especially during the routine practical work of the pathology department. In addition, the afterbirth is not always examined histologically, especially in cases where there is no information about TB in a woman in labor or maternity at the time of delivery. In addition, often for a routine histological examination of the placenta, a minimum amount of material is often taken with the preparation of only a few sections from each block (usually 1–2 sections). We agree with the opinion of the authors, who insist on mandatory histobacterioscopic examination of the placenta to identify acid-resistant bacteria in the study of afterbirth and fetuses from women suffering from TB. In addition to histobacterioscopy with Ziehl-Neelsen staining, we use IHC examination with tuberculosis antibodies, as well as molecular biological examination of placental fragments (PCR examination to detect MBT DNA). These studies are especially important in cases of HIV-associated tuberculosis in a pregnant woman. There are indications of the detection of acid-resistant bacteria in fetal vessels, interstitial fibrin and septa. A case of detection of a variety of acid-resistant bacteria in the villous tissue of abortive material in a patient receiving therapy for destructive pulmonary tuberculosis, while necrosis and granulomatous reaction in the endometrium were not detected. In our studies, the pathogen was detected histobacterioscopically and immunohistochemically in the site of granulomatous inflammation of the placenta (in necrotic confluent granuloma) and in a large focus of caseous necrosis. In one case, MBT DNA was found in a randomly taken placental site in the absence of signs of tuberculous inflammation in the afterbirth and with negative results of Ziehl-Neelsen histobacterioscopy (subsequently, the presence of generalized tuberculosis with tuberculous endometritis in the mother and generalized tuberculosis in the newborn was established).

Cases of tuberculous lesions of the placenta with multiple tuberculous rashes, including necrosis without giant cells in the decidual tissue, multiple granulomas in the interstitial space and in the villi, chorion was poorly involved. The previously stated assumption about the resistance of syncytium to mycobacterial infection was subsequently revised after the detection of necrotic changes in the trophoblast.

Currently, congenital tuberculosis is quite rare, and sick infants are cured in most cases. It is noted that if the placenta is affected by tuberculous inflammation, the child may be healthy. Thus, a case of placenta examination (Plac. membranacea) at 35 weeks of gestation from a patient with tuberculous peritonitis, with the detection of tuberculous granulomas in the placental site, is described, but the child is healthy.

Thus, tuberculous lesions of the placenta and fetus are more likely to develop with generalized miliary progressive tuberculosis in the mother. The volume of damage to the placenta can be different. All elements of the afterbirth may be involved in the pathological process. It is characterized by a weak development of granulomatous inflammation elements with a predominance of alterative and exudative tissue reactions, involvement of placental vessels in the process. The pathway of infection of the placenta is usually hematogenous, although a descending pathway or a mixed pathway of infection is also possible. The ways of infection of the fetus/newborn can also be different and a mixed path of infection is also possible. Morphological differential diagnosis should be carried out primarily with syphilis, mycotic lesions, leprosy, listeriosis. Tuberculous damage to the placenta does not always mean the development of tuberculosis in a child.

Macroscopic examination does not always reveal any changes characteristic of TB. To detect tuberculosis of the placenta, it is necessary to histologically examine a large number of fragments taken from various parts of the placenta/placenta with serial sections, conduct histobacterioscopy according to Ziehl-Neelsen to identify acid-resistant bacteria, IHC examination with tuberculosis antibodies to determine mycobacteria, conduct a molecular biological study (in particular, PCR examination of the native placenta/placenta material or material from histological paraffin blocks in order to identify M. tuberculosis DNA). It is necessary to conduct a complex morphological study from women with TB or who have previously suffered TB, since tuberculous inflammation in the placenta may have minimal or atypical manifestations with erasure or absence of a granulomatous reaction, manifested by "non-specific" reactions. Routine microscopic examination may not be enough. Our experience convinces us of the application of the above-mentioned comprehensive examination of the afterbirth for early diagnostics or prevention of the development of TB in a child born from a mother with tuberculosis.

Current diagnostic criteria for congenital TB include a proven tuberculous lesion in the neonate and at least one of the following: lesions in the first week of life, a primary hepatic TB complex or caseating hepatic granulomas (due to transmission through the umbilical vein, hence, forming a primary TB complex in the fetal liver),

TB of the placenta or maternal genital tract, or exclusion of postnatal transmission.

Clinical Examples

Patient A with infiltrative pulmonary TB received anti-tuberculosis therapy. The delivery is timely, with a full-term fetus. The child is healthy.

Micro description of the placenta

The placenta corresponds to the third trimester of pregnancy, full-term pregnancy. Moderate circulatory disorders in the form of fullness of villous capillaries, there are areas of erythrocyte stasis in the interstitial space. Small calcinates in small amounts. Moderate signs of chronic placental insufficiency with compensatory phenomena. This was manifested by a small number of capillaries in the part of terminal villi or a sufficient number of capillaries with a small number of syncytio-capillary membranes formed, a small number of syncytial nodules. At the same time, terminal villi with signs of angiomatosis and areas of syncytial nodule proliferation were detected.

Several single and fused epithelioid giant cell granulomas were found, granulomas without signs of organization. Were noted merging granulomas (Fig. 5.7 Patient A) with a necrosis site and leukocytes in the center, without signs of fibrosis. There is a fine calcinate in the center of the necrotic masses. However, given the active granulomatous inflammation, this calcinate should not be regarded as a manifestation of the organization in the area of tuberculous inflammation.

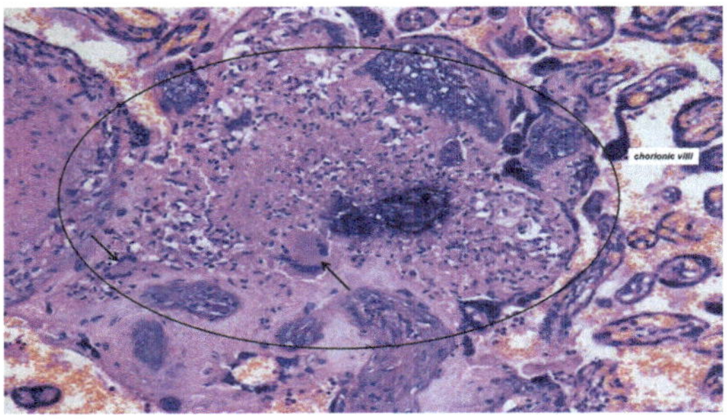

Fig. 5.7 Patient A. Placenta. Tuberculosis of the placenta. Merging granulomas with necrosis in the center (the granuloma is shown by an oval frame, giant multinucleated Langhans cells are indicated by arrows). H-E. ×200

Probably, the granulomatous infectious process developed in the area of localization of one of the calcifications of the placenta, the presence of which is quite common in full-term pregnancy.

The umbilical cord has no signs of inflammation both at the fetal end and at the place of attachment to the placenta. The membranes are without signs of inflammation.

Patient R., 28 years old with generalized TB, with lesions of the lungs, pleura, brain, mammary glands, placenta. Reactivation during the second pregnancy of previously diagnosed and cured tuberculous pleurisy (a socially safe patient from a prosperous family with good income, working, committed to treatment). The child born from the second pregnancy died of congenital generalized tuberculosis, which was confirmed by the results of an autopsy study with histological examination of all organs, histobacterioscopy according to Ziehl-Neelsen, as well as a molecular biological method with PCR examination of the material from the paraffin blocks of the affected organs with the detection of MBT DNA [89].

The biopsy of pleura was performed during pregnancy contains fragments of a thickened pleura due to fibrosis, sometimes lined with mesothelium with reactive changes. In the thickness of the fibrotic pleura, there is an unevenly pronounced diffuse lymphoid infiltration, as well as multiple epithelioid giant cell granulomas, both single and merging. There are single granulomas with a necrosis in the center. Granulomas of various ages: thin loose single collagen fibers around individual granulomas, there are also small forming granulomas (Fig. 5.8 Patient R1).

MBT DNA was isolated in the pleural fluid as well as in the native material.

In the excised area of the breast (biopsy in the postpartum period), there is unevenly pronounced edema, weakly and moderately pronounced lymphoid infiltration, sometimes with an admixture of leukocytes. There is moderate fibrosis and mild lymphoid infiltration around part of the ducts. Parts of the ducts are dilated, proliferation of epithelial cells, epithelial cells are enlarged, with enlarged pits, vacuolization of the cytoplasm, cells of the "colostrum" type. These epithelial changes were regarded as lactation

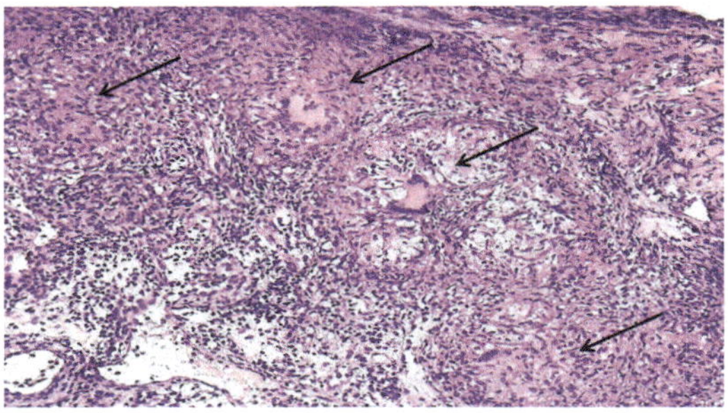

Fig. 5.8 Patient R. Pleura. Tuberculous pleurisy. Lymphoid infiltration and multiple granulomas in the fibrotic pleura (granulomas are indicated by arrows). H-E. ×200

(biopsy was performed in the postpartum period). However, significant desquamation of the epithelium, the presence of inter- and intraepithelial leukocytes attracted attention. Also, necrotic eosinophilic structureless masses and a large number of leukocytes were observed in the lumen of the ducts among desquamated epithelial cells with vacuolization of the cytoplasm and "colostrum bodies." No signs of granulomatous inflammation were found. Histobacterioscopy according to Ziehl-Neelsen revealed acid-resistant bacteria in the contents of the ducts of the breast, which were identified as mycobacteria during IHC examination with antibodies to M. tuberculosis. During the PCR examination of the breast material from the paraffin block, the DNA of Mycobacterium tuberculosis was determined. Thus, on the basis of a comprehensive study, tuberculous mastitis, an active process, was established (Fig. 5.9a–c)

The placenta corresponds to the third trimester of pregnancy, full-term pregnancy. Moderate circulatory disorders with the formation of an ischemic infarction in the thickness of the placenta, with the presence of single necrotic chorionic villi, partially thrombosed vessel and with weakly/moderately pronounced reactive inflammation in the form of uneven diffuse focal leukocyte infiltration along the periphery of the infarction site (Fig. 5.10). No acid-resistant bacteria were found in the area of ischemic infarction during the Ziehl-Neelsen staining. No MBT DNA was detected during PCR examination of a placental fragment from the infarction site.

In one of the fragments of the placenta, outside of the above-described ischemic infarction, a single rounded focus of necrosis was detected. In the perifocal areas of the placenta, there was a fullness of the interstitial space, as well as moderate edema and fullness of the vessels of the adjacent villi. Leukocyte infiltration was detected in necrotic masses in the center, there were no signs of granulomatous inflammation, including epithelioid and giant multinucleated cells of the Langhans type (Fig. 5.10 Patient R5). Histobacterioscopic examination with Ziehl-Neelsen staining was performed with the identification of acid-resistant bacteria in the microarray of necrosis. During PCR examination of placental material from a paraffin block taken in the area of the military necrotic site, MBT DNA was found.

No signs of inflammation were found in the umbilical cord, a section of the fetal part of the umbilical cord and a section of the umbilical cord from the area of attachment to the placenta were examined. No signs of inflammation were found in the fetal membranes.

In this case, the infection of the child could occur hematogenously, transplacentally, which is confirmed by clinical data and the results of an autopsy examination with the detection of damage to the liver, spleen and subhepatic lymph nodes, the rapid development of the tuberculosis process and massive generalization.

However, it is impossible to exclude the simultaneous possibility of infection by aspiration or ingestion of infected amniotic fluid, as well as during breastfeeding (since the woman has tuberculosis mastitis).

Patient G., 19 years old, had not previously suffered from TB, socially well-off, from a family with little income, all family members are working, family relations are friendly, the child is welcome. TB was detected 2 months after childbirth during emergency hospitalization in a general medical network with a clinic for abdominal cavity catastrophe, perforation of a hollow organ. Signs of active tuberculous inflammation were found in the surgical material of the perforated ileum. Subsequently, it was found out that the woman was in periodic family contact with her

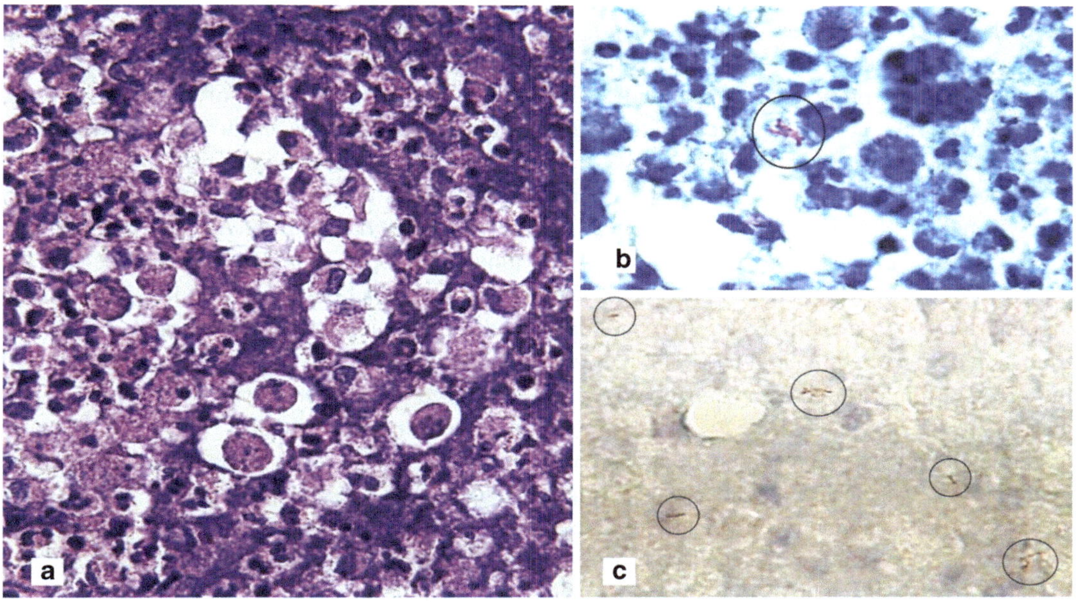

Fig. 5.9 Patient R (3). Mammary gland. Tuberculous mastitis. (**a**) the contents of the lumen of the breast duct—desquamated epithelial cells, "colostrum cells," a fragment of the previous figure in purulent necrotic exudate; (**b**) acid-resistant bacteria in purulent necrotic contents of the breast duct (in a round frame); (**c**) mycobacteria in purulent necrotic contents of the breast duct (in a round frame). (a) H-E; (b) Ziehl-Neelsen staining; (c) IHC with antibodies to M. tuberculosis

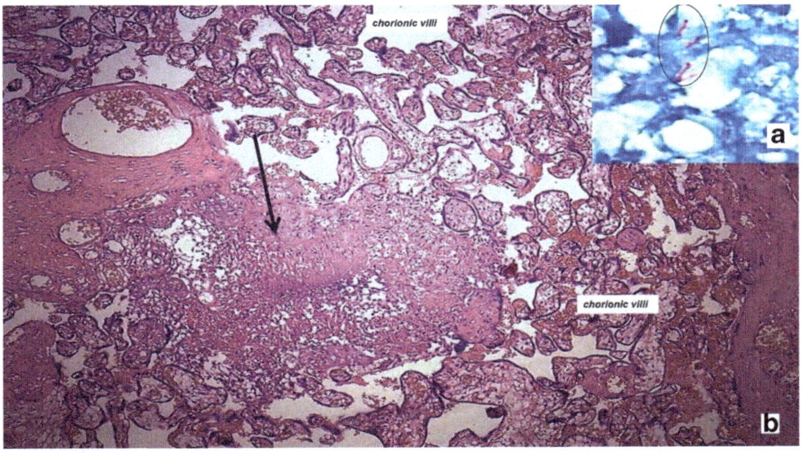

Fig. 5.10 Patient R (5). Placenta. Tuberculosis of the placenta. Miliary necrotic lesion with leukocyte infiltration (indicated by an arrow). In the inset "b," acid-resistant bacteria in this hearth (in an oval frame, colored red). (a) Staining with hematoxylin and eosin, ×100; (b) Cyl-Nielsen staining, ×1000. During PCR examination of the placenta material from the paraffin block, MBT DNA was detected

brother, a tuberculosis patient who lived in another city. Tuberculosis in her brother was detected as a result of an epidemiological investigation of contacts after the death of patient G. The woman died on the 6th day after hospitalization, from generalized tuberculosis with damage to the lungs, kidneys, spleen, adrenal glands, intestines, lymph nodes (confirmed histologically, histobacterioscopically with Ziehl-Neelsen staining and molecular biological method—PCR examination of pieces of organs from paraffin blocks, MBT DNA detected). The placenta was not presented for the study. The child is alive, tuberculosis has not been detected, and was under the control of phthisiologists.

A uterus with a neck of 10 × 5.4 × 3 cm, flabby; a neck with a slit-like throat, the so-called "giving birth." The uterus is without nodules, the thickness of the uterine walls is about 1 cm. The myometrium is grayish-pinkish, the endometrium is red, in the right lateral parts of the uterus the endometrium is rough with whitish-yellowish overlays.

Subinvolutionary changes, large vessels with hyalinized walls, clusters of siderophages, and weak signs of endometrial regeneration were found in the uterus in the placental bed. Also in the area of the placental bed, there are small encapsulated and hyalinized foci of necrosis, areas of necrosis without signs of organization and single and merging epithelioid cell granulomas, and single scattered giant Langhans cells. Single acid-resistant bacteria were detected in the areas of granulomatous inflammation during Ziehl-Neelsen staining (Fig. 5.11 Patient G1).

In the preserved areas of the endometrium, pronounced hemorrhages, diffuse lymphoid infiltration with an admixture of histiocytes, plasmocytes, leukocytes (subacute endometritis), acid-resistant bacteria were not found during histobacterioscopy according to Ziehl-Neelsen, but small accumulations of non-acid-resistant coccal and bacillary microflora were found.

Confluent fuzzy granulomas and isolated organized foci of necrosis were found in the myometrium and perimetry.

Thus, tuberculous subacute panmetritis occurs, including the development of the tuberculous process in the placental bed. Single acid-resistant bacteria were detected in the placental bed area during Ziehl-Neelsen histobacterioscopy. DNA of MBT was detected in the placental bed material (the material from the paraffin block was examined, a piece of tissue was taken from the site of granulomatous inflammation and the second fragment from the site of necrosis.

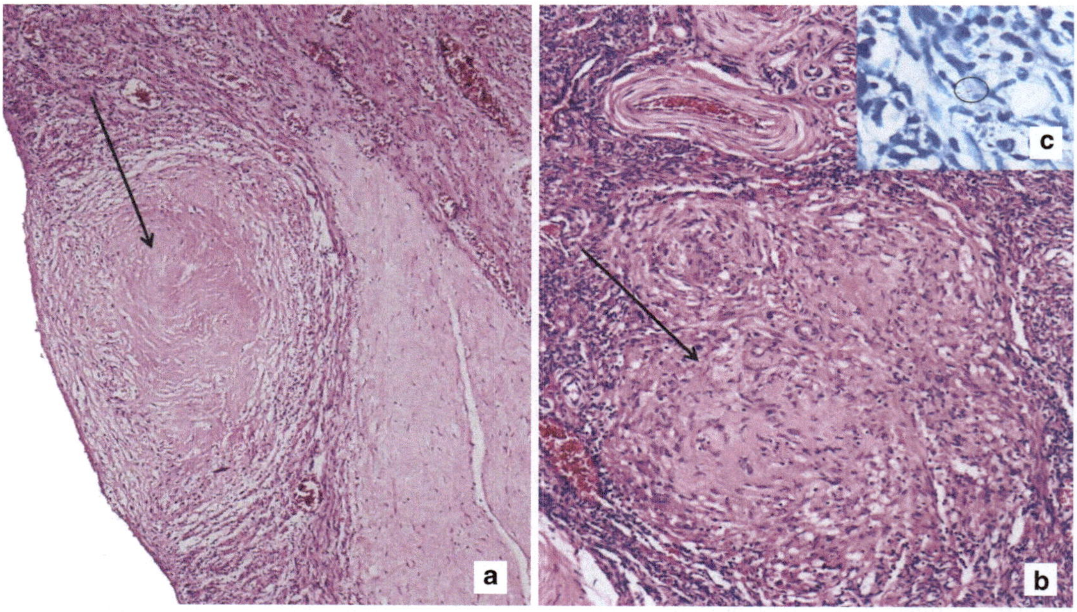

Fig. 5.11 Patient G (1). Uterus. The placental bed. Tuberculous inflammation of a subacute nature in the area of the placental bed is an encapsulated focus of necrosis without signs of activity of the tuberculous process (**a**, indicated by an arrow); merging granulomas (**b**, indicated by an arrow), on the inset "c" an acid-resistant bacterium in the material from the placental bed (in a round frame, colored red). (a, b) H-E, ×100; (c) Ziehl-Neelsen staining, ×1000. During PCR examination of the placental bed material from the paraffin block, MBT DNA was found

Pathological diagnosis

Generalized miliary tuberculosis in the progressive phase with damage to the lungs (in bronchoalveolar lavage, DNA MBT was found in vivo), liver, spleen, adrenal glands, kidneys (miliary tuberculosis of the kidneys + caseous papillitis of the left kidney), peritoneum, intestines (infiltrative ulcerative tuberculosis of the ileum and caecum), intestinal mesentery, lymph nodes (intra-thoracic, mesenteric), uterus (tuberculous miliary panmetritis, including tuberculous inflammation in the placental bed, MBT DNA detected).

Complications: Perforation of tuberculous intestinal ulcers. Serous fibrinous peritonitis. Polysegmental bacterial fibrinous-purulent pneumonia with microabsorption (histobacterioscopically predominantly Gram-positive coccal flora). Subacute epicarditis and interstitial myocarditis, secondary metabolic damage to cardiomyocytes. Liquid blood in the cavities of the heart and large vessels. Pulmonary edema. Diffuse alveolar lung injury with the formation of hyaline membranes. DIC syndrome—fibrin-erythrocyte thrombi in the microvascular bed, microbleeds in the lungs, endometrium, myocardium, omentum, gastric mucosa, small intestine, calyx-pelvic kidney system; micronecrosis of the pancreas, adrenal glands, focal necrosis of the epithelium of the renal tubules; acute erosion of the gastric mucosa. Anemia, thrombocytopenia, coagulopathy, hepatic-renal insufficiency. Swelling of the brain.

Concomitant diseases: 78 days after timely delivery in head presentation, fetal hypotrophy (postpartum uterine subinvolution).

Operations:

1. Diagnostic laparoscopy.
2. Laparotomy, resection of the iliac and dome of the cecum. Nasointestinal intubation. Drainage of the abdominal cavity.
3. Relaparotomy, formation of entero-transverse anastomosis "side-to-side," abdominal drainage.

Patient W., HIV infection, stage 4B. Spontaneous miscarriage at the age of 18–19 weeks of pregnancy, vacuum extraction of the fetus. HIV infection was detected during hospitalization for miscarriage, the woman did not know about her HIV infection, was not been previously examined. The elder child is 8 years old, has been ill for a long time and is often ill, has not previously been tested for HIV infection. Tuberculosis in a woman was detected during her lifetime, during an examination after HIV infection was established. The previous fluorographic examination of the lungs 3 years ago, without pathology. She died 7 days after a spontaneous miscarriage. Death followed from HIV infection in AIDS stage, a phase of progression outside of antiretroviral therapy, with the presence as a secondary disease of acute general miliary tuberculosis with lesions of the lungs, intratoracic and intra-abdominal lymph nodes, red bone marrow, kidneys, spleen, liver, uterus, fallopian tubes, placenta, peritoneum, brain the brain. Cytomegalovirus lung damage was also detected.

The placenta corresponds to the second trimester of pregnancy, immature intermediate villi predominate, mature intermediate villi are present, terminal villi are not formed. Uneven partial fibrosis of the villi. There are areas of the placenta with necrotized chorionic villi surrounded by fibrinoid. Foci of caseous necrosis with leukocyte infiltration were detected in the depth of the placenta, a layer of "specific" granulation tissue was not formed along the periphery of the necrotic masses. There are no granulomas, as well as individual cellular elements of granulomatous inflammation—epithelioid cells and giant multinucleated cells of the Langhans type and the type of foreign bodies have not been identified. No signs of organization were found in the foci of necrosis, no signs of encapsulation of necrotic foci, no collagen fibers in necrotic masses. Acid-resistant bacteria were detected in necrotic masses during Ziehl-Neelsen staining (Fig. 5.12 Patient W1). During PCR examination of the placenta material from paraffin blocks (site with necrotic focus), mycobacterium tuberculosis complex DNA was detected.

The basal lamina had focal polymorphocellular infiltration from lymphoid cells, macrophages, plasma cells, and neutrophilic leukocytes, which was regarded as a manifestation of subacute basal deciduitis.

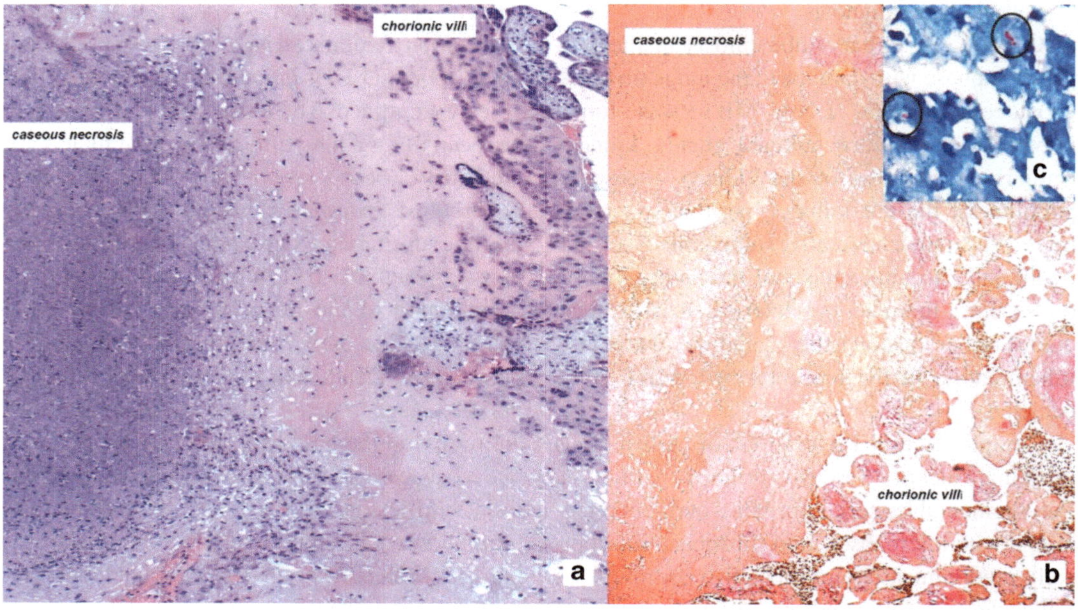

Fig. 5.12 Patient W (1). Placenta. Tuberculous caseous placentitis. (**a**) A focus of necrosis with uneven leukocyte infiltration, with the absence of elements of granulomatous inflammation; (**b**) no signs of organization in the focus of necrosis, no formation of a fibrous capsule around the necrotic focus was detected, no collagen fibers in necrotic masses; (**c**) acid-resistant bacteria in necrotic masses (in a round frame, colored red). (a) H-E, ×100; (b) van Gieson staining, ×40; (c) Ziehl-Neelsen staining, ×1000

Umbilical cord without significant changes. Histological examination of the fetal membranes revealed signs of focal subacute chorionamnionitis: focal polymorphocellular infiltration localized mainly in the chorial plate.

The uterus has a flabby elastic consistency, triangular shape, 13 × 8 × 7 cm, with a gray-red surface. On the serous membrane in the projection of the ampoule of the fallopian tubes with a transition to a wide ligament of the uterus, yellow-white tubercular rashes, miliary and small focal with a diameter of up to 0.4 cm. Fallopian tubes are unevenly thickened, deformed due to adhesions, with injected full-blooded vessels on the surface, multiple miliary rashes (Fig. 5.13 Patient W2). There are whitish structureless masses on the incision in the lumen of the pipe, when they are removed, it is established that the mucous membrane is destroyed. Ovaries are ovoid in shape, 1.8 × 1.4 × 1.0 cm each, of a tightly elastic consistency, gray-white in color. The cervix is edematous, hyperemic, flabby consistency, the external pharynx is rounded, 0.7 cm in diameter. There are traces of red loose blood coagulations in the cervical canal, the mucous membrane is gray-pink in color, with single Nabothian cysts. The uterine cavity is expanded, the wall thickness in the bottom area is 2.5 cm, in the lower segment up to 2.0 cm. The endometrium is loose, brownish-red in color. In the uterine cavity, on the back wall, with a spread to the bottom, there is a mixed blood bundle 11.0 × 7.0 × 1.0 cm. Upon separation of this convolution, a red-brown area with a rough surface, sometimes covered with delicate fibrin films, was revealed on a spongy-looking incision (Fig. 5.14 Patient W3 a,b).

In the myometrium of the posterior wall of the uterus with a transition to the right wall, isthmic department and bottom, vascular fullness, mixed blood clots, focal lymphocytic infiltration, indistinct strands of epithelioid cells without granuloma formation are noted. Extensive areas of endometrial destruction with its replacement by caseous-necrotic masses with leukocyte infiltration. There is pronounced polymorphocellular infiltration in the endometrium, areas of "specific" granulation tissue with indistinct epi-

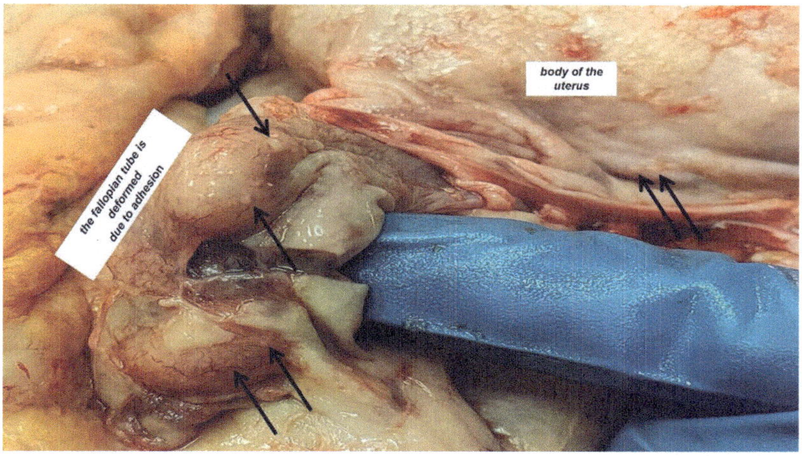

Fig. 5.13 Patient W (2). Uterus with appendages. Tuberculous tuberculous rashes in the perimetry and on the surface of the fallopian tubes (indicated by arrows). An unfixed macropreparation

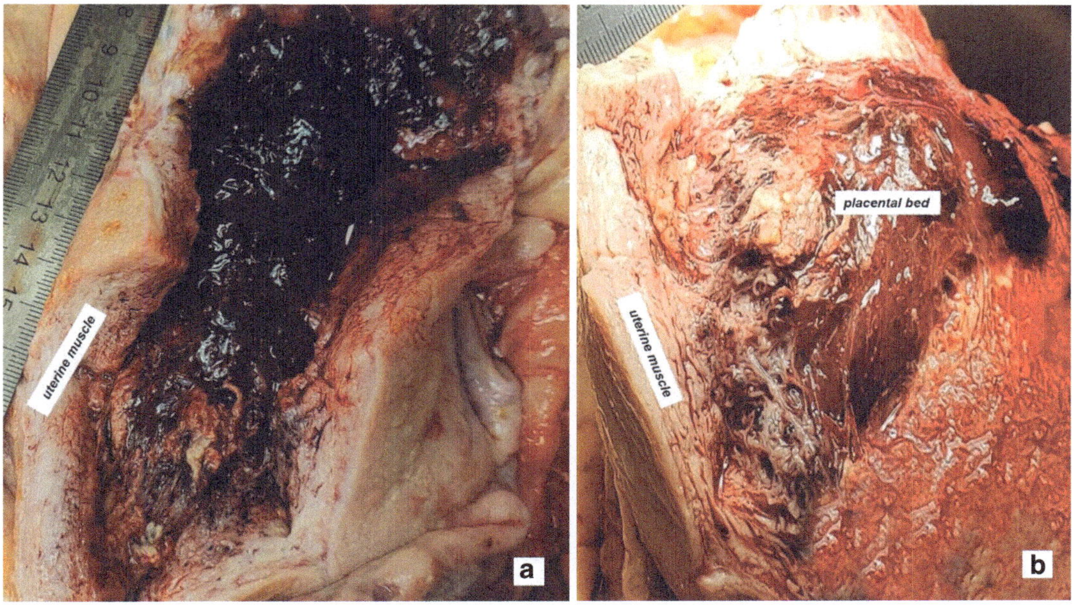

Fig. 5.14 Patient W (3). Uterus. (**a**) dissected uterus, blood coagulation in the placental bed area; (**b**) dissected uterus, placental bed area (blood coagulation removed)—the placental bed is covered with fibrin. Unfixed macropreparations

thelioid cell granulomas with single giant Langhans cells. The endometrial glands are dilated, and there is mucus with leukocytes in their lumen. There are elements of trophoblast. Acid-resistant bacteria were found in necrotic masses during staining by the Ziehl-Neelsen method. PCR examination of uterine sections from the placental bed (native material and material from the paraffin block) revealed the Mycobacterium tuberculosis complex (Fig. 5.15 Patient W4 a,b).

In the fallopian tubes, fibrin overlays on the serous membrane and multiple purulent-necrotic foci without signs of granuloma formation (macroscopically tubercular rashes on the surface of the fallopian tubes). There are multiple necrotic and purulent necrotic focuses in the serous layer and muscle layers. The mucous membrane of the fallopian tubes is destroyed and replaced by caseous necrotic masses. The lumen of the tubes is filled by caseous masses, in which single epithelioid cells have been identified. These changes

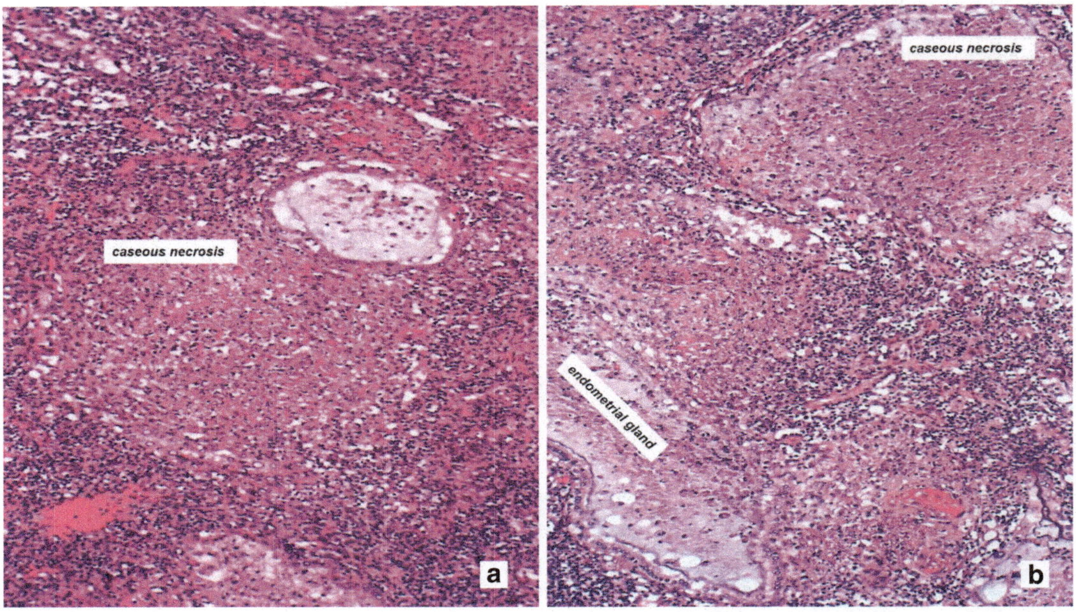

Fig. 5.15 Patient W (4). Uterus. The placental bed. Tuberculous inflammation in the placental bed, an active process. Purulent necrotic foci without epithelioid giant cell reaction along the periphery, without signs of organization. There are no signs of granulomatous inflammation. Histobacterioscopy with Ziehl-Neelsen staining revealed acid-resistant bacteria. PCR examination of the placental bed material (from the paraffin block) revealed MBT DNA.H-E. ×100

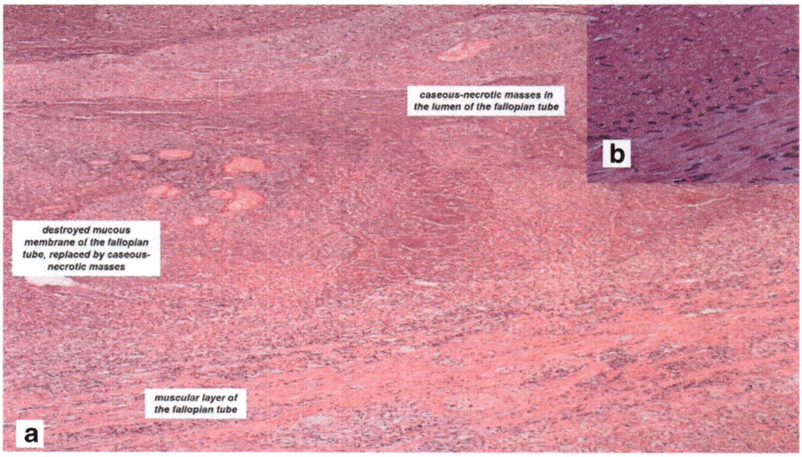

Fig. 5.16 Patient W (5). Fallopian tube. Caseous salpingitis. (**a**) The destroyed mucous membrane of the tube, replaced by caseous-necrotic masses. The lumen of the fallopian tube is lined with caseous masses; (**b**) A fragment of (**a**) necrotic masses with single epithelioid cells in the lumen of the fallopian tube. H-E (a) ×100; (b) ×200.

were regarded as tuberculous caseous pansalpingitis (Fig. 5.16 Patient W5 a,b). Acid-resistant bacteria were found in the necrotic masses of tubercular eruptions and in the lumen of the fallopian tube when stained according to Ziehl-Neelsen. A PCR examination of a section of the fallopian tube with necrotic masses revealed the DNA of Mycobacterium tuberculosis complex.

Pathological diagnosis

HIV infection, AIDS, progression phase outside of antiretroviral therapy (immune status: CD4+ 130 cl/mcl (34%), CD8+ 153 cl/mcl (41%), CD4/CD8—0.85), with late spontaneous incomplete miscarriage at 18–19 weeks of pregnancy. Vacuum aspiration of the contents of the uterine cavity.

Secondary diseases:

1. Generalized tuberculosis in the progressive phase, with lung damage (MBT DNA "+" in vivo in bronchoalveolar lavage), red bone marrow, kidneys, spleen, liver, peritoneum (miliary dissemination), brain (tuberculous leptomeningitis, autopsy PCR examination of cerebrospinal fluid—M. tuberculosis complete DNA was detected, low concentration), intratoracic lymph nodes, mesenteric, subhepatic, parapancreatic lymph nodes (caseous lymphadenitis), uterus (caseous endometritis), fallopian tubes (caseous pansalpingitis), tuberculous caseous placentitis.

   Ziehl-Neelsen histobacterioscopy allowed to detect acid-resistant bacteria in the foci of caseous necrosis of all organs. During PCR examination of native material and tissue sections from paraffin blocks of various internal organs, including lungs, placenta, uterus, peritoneum, fallopian tubes, MBT DNA was found.
2. Cytomegalovirus infection with lung damage (cells with cytomegalic transformation were found in the lungs, lifetime detection of Cytomegalovirus DNA in the blood).

Complications: Pulmonary edema. Swelling of the brain. Bilateral hydrothorax (500 ml each). Splenomegaly (spleen weight 745 g). DIC syndrome: subpleural and subepicardial hemorrhages in the conjunctiva; fibrin and fibrin-erythrocyte thrombi in the vessels of the microcirculatory bed of internal organs; focal necrosis of the adrenal glands, necronephrosis. Anemia, thrombocytopenia, coagulopathy.

In this observation, it can be stated that severe tuberculous alterative lesion of the placenta and uterus with appendages led to miscarriage at 18–19 weeks of pregnancy (it was not possible to conduct a morphological examination of the fetus for the presence of congenital tuberculosis). The woman died of HIV-associated generalized tuberculosis. Histological examination revealed signs of acute progression of tuberculosis with the development of purulent-necrotic lesions in many organs with a large number of acid-resistant bacteria, the absence of the formation of a productive granulomatous reaction in conditions of severe immune deficiency and the absence of signs of the organization of foci of inflammation.

Patient T., 25 years old has not been ill with TB before, denies contact with a tuberculosis patient. The first pregnancy 3 years ago, cesarean section, baby weight 3440 g, height 53 cm. During the second pregnancy at the age of 20 weeks, she noted a single rise in temperature to 39 °C during the day, pain in the right half of the chest. Ultrasound and X-ray examination of the chest organs were not performed during pregnancy. Second delivery timely operative abdominal delivery (cesarean section), baby weight 3420 g, height 52 cm, Apgar score 8/9 points, screamed immediately. She was discharged home, breastfed the baby. Seven days after giving birth, febrile fever, weakness, and headache appeared. She was hospitalized in an emergency. Computed tomography of the chest revealed dissemination in the lungs, right-sided hydrothorax with leakage into the interstitial crevices. Tuberculosis of the lungs was suspected, in connection with which the woman was hospitalized in a maternity hospital at the city tuberculosis control center. As a result of a comprehensive examination, generalized TB was established in the progressive phase with damage to the lungs, pleura, brain, peripheral lymph nodes, uterus (tuberculous metroendometritis); Mycobacterium tuberculosis complex DNA was found in sputum, aspirate from the uterine cavity, placenta. The patient received anti-tuberculosis therapy.

The child from the second pregnancy was not vaccinated with BCG (mother's refusal), was attached to the breast from the first day after birth, was breastfed for 8 days. A month after birth, he was admitted to a children's hospital with febrile fever and signs of acute respiratory illness. During the examination, the reaction to the Mantoux test is negative, the blood test for MBT by the T-SPOT method was negative. Mycobacterium tuberculosis complex DNA was found in a pharyngeal swab. Computed tomography revealed dissemination in the lungs, signs of pathological contents in the cells of the mastoid process and tympanic cavity on the right, hepatosplenomegaly, multiple hypodensal foci in the liver and spleen, conglomerate of lymph nodes in the area of the liver gate and head of the pancreas, cholecystocholangitis, pileflebitis. There is lymphocytic cytosis in the cerebrospinal fluid. Laboratory studies have shown signs of a systemic inflammatory reaction, leukocytosis with a shift of the leukocyte formula to the left, coagulopathy (a sharp increase in the level of D-dimer), liver failure. The child in serious condition was transferred for treatment to the children's intensive care unit in special hospital Diagnosis: Generalized tuberculosis in the progressive phase with damage to the lungs, liver, spleen, brain, intra-thoracic and intra-abdominal lymph nodes, middle ear on the right, right-sided tuberculous mastoiditis.

The father of the children and the elder child were examined by an outpatient phthisiologist, tuberculosis was not detected.

Placenta corresponds to full-term pregnancy. Focal circulatory disorders in the form of small hemorrhages in the interstitial space, in the subcellular areas; moderate edema of individual intermediate chorionic villi is noted. There are signs of increased vascular permeability of several intermediate villi in the form of edema, plasma impregnation of the vascular wall. Signs of minimal productive vasculitis were found in single vessels of intermediate villi. There are small "old" placental infarctions.

Changes indicating the presence of chronic placental insufficiency with compensation phenomena were revealed (part of terminal villi with a small number of capillaries, syncytio-capillary membranes and syncytial kidneys; part of villi with signs of angiomatosis, focal proliferation of syncytial kidneys).

No signs of basal deciduitis, inflammation in the umbilical cord and fetal membranes were found.

There were no changes in the placenta characteristic of tuberculous lesions. Acid-resistant bacteria were not detected during Ziehl-Neelsen histobacterioscopy. The placenta material from the paraffin block was sent for PCR examination, in which the DNA of M. tuberculosis complete was detected.

The aspirate from the uterine cavity is represented by mucus with leukocytes and small areas of the endometrium. Endometrium with signs of reverse development (1.5 months after delivery), endometrial glands of proliferative type. In the stroma of the endometrium there is a rather dense infiltrate of lymphocytes, plasma cells, with an admixture of leukocytes. There are single very small, indistinct macrophage-epithelioid granulomas forming in the stroma of the endometrium. Small foci of caseous necrosis with leukocyte infiltration and a weakly expressed epithelioid cell reaction along the edge were also revealed.

M. tuberculosis complete DNA was found in the native aspirate material from the uterine cavity.

This case has clinical value for several reasons. There were no signs of tuberculous inflammation in the placenta, but a PCR examination of paraffin block material from placenta revealed MBT DNA, which suggests an intrauterine, transplacental route of infection. The presence of pileflebitis, liver and spleen damage, tuberculous lymphadenitis of the lymph nodes of the liver gate, massive infection of the child and rapid generalization of tuberculosis also indicate in favor of this pathway of infection. In the case of hematogenic infection, Mycobacterium tuberculosis penetrates through the umbilical vein, the umbilical vein into the fetal liver, the lymph nodes of the liver gate, into the inferior vena cava with further generalization of TB. Damage to the liver and lymph nodes of the liver gate (caseous lymphadenitis) is considered the main sign of congenital tuberculosis.

In addition, taking in consideration the close contact with a mother with TB (with possible bacterial excretion with sputum and discharge from the genital tract), airborne infection is also possible.

Breastfeeding as a possible way of infecting a child also cannot be excluded.

5.2.4 Chlamydiosis

All chlamydia—representatives of the Chlamydia family—are obligate intracellular microorganisms of humans and animals, widely distributed in nature. Dangerous to humans are Chlamydia trachomatis (Ch. trachomatis)—sexually transmitted, household contact and vertical pathways, Chlamydia pneumoniae (Ch. pneumoniae)—airborne, and *Chlamydophila psittaci* (*Ch. psittaci*)—airborne and, rarely, alimentary. The biological properties and features of the existence of chlamydia are of the same type and are covered in detail in the literature.

Chlamydia are unable to synthesize ATP, GTP, and a number of enzymatic systems. They can exist in different forms (stages of development), of which elementary and reticular corpuscles are the most studied. The elementary body penetrates into the host cell by adsorption endocytosis, is filtered through bacterial filters and does not grow on artificial nutrient media, unlike other bacteria. The reticular body, the reproductive form of intracellular existence, has the structure of a typical Gr (−) bacterium. Against the background of a deficiency of metabolites necessary for the development of the bacterium or with inadequate mechanisms of protection of the host cell, the pathogen persists. The interaction of the infectious agent with the host cell is diverse (reproduction, persistence with the development of aberrant reticular bodies and reactivation,), in addition, depending on the conditions and form of existence of the pathogen, inhibition or activation of apoptosis of host cells is noted. Chlamydia can be found practically in all type of cells, disrupt phagocytosis, spreading as part of these cells throughout the body, and possess antigenic "mimicry."

5.2.4.1 Lesions of the Afterbirth in Chlamydia

For the first time, isolated chlamydia from 22 afterbirth during artificial abortions and by injecting isolated pathogens into pregnant cows, he received severe placentitis leading to spontaneous miscarriages. Later, Wilt (1976) systematically examining the afterbirth of women living in endemic foci of chlamydia in Northern Canada, also isolated this pathogen. Zinserling reports on the possibility of intrauterine chlamydia in humans. He believes that infection is more likely to occur intranatally when passing through the birth canal. However, he also describes a case of chlamydia at birth by cesarean section. Alexander and Harrison and Martins note a fairly high frequency (2–4%) of infection of pregnant women with chlamydia, the presence of cervicitis. On average, 26% of children born are also infected: they have conjunctivitis and pneumonia.

In the work of Altschuler, when examining 100 sequences in 30, chorioamnionitis was found, presumably of a chlamydial nature.

Structural changes characteristic of chlamydia were also observed in vascular endothelium, amniocytes, decidual and trophoblastic cells of the basal lamina, smooth and villous chorion in the form of fine vacuolization of the cytoplasm and the presence of small basophilic and pas-positive inclusions and Galberstedter-Provacek bodies in vacuoles (Fig. 5.17). In addition, vascular disorders of varying severity, various variants of pathological immaturity were observed in the afterbirth, which led to placental insufficiency, including acute in 14, chronic compensated in 13, chronic subcompensated in 3. This allowed us to determine the degree of risk for possible pathology of the newborn.

Most recently, we conducted a study of the outcomes of women suffering from preeclampsia against the background of a new coronavirus infection. Along with immaturity with signs of dissociated maturation, signs of infectious lesions were revealed. Along with the non-constant detection of SARSCOVID-2 s-antigen in all placental membranes, a significant number of extracellular and intracellular pas-positive corpuscles and a distinct positive immunohistochemical reaction with serum to Chlamydia trachomatis (Figs. 5.18 and 5.19) were naturally detected. Many aspects of the revealed phenomenon need further study.

5.2.4.2 Intrauterine Chlamydiosis

The significant frequency and great clinical significance of intrauterine chlamydia is currently recognized by all the numerous researchers discussing the issue of perinatal infections. There is evidence that at least 6–7% of children may be

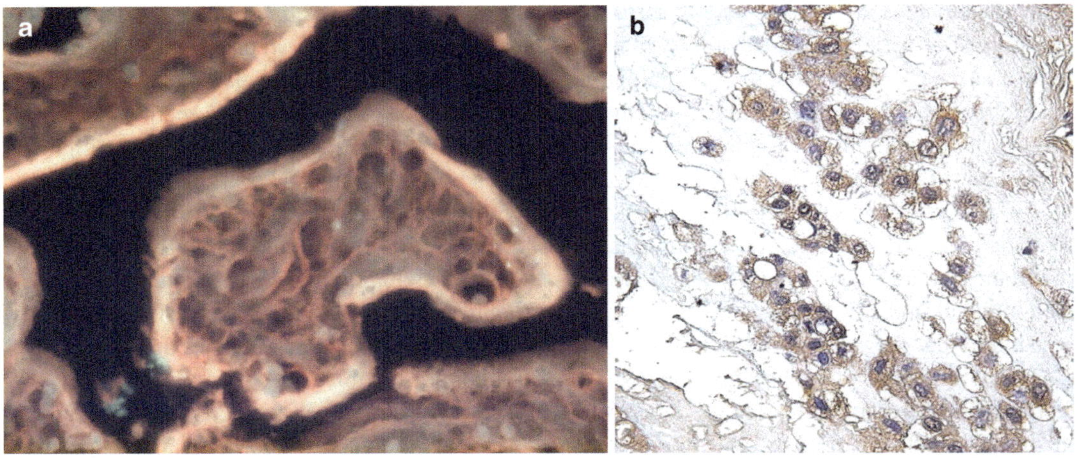

Fig. 5.17 (**a**) Chlamydia antigen in stem villus. Immunofluorescent microscopy/×600. (**b**) Chlamydia trachomatis antigen in decidua. IHC/×600

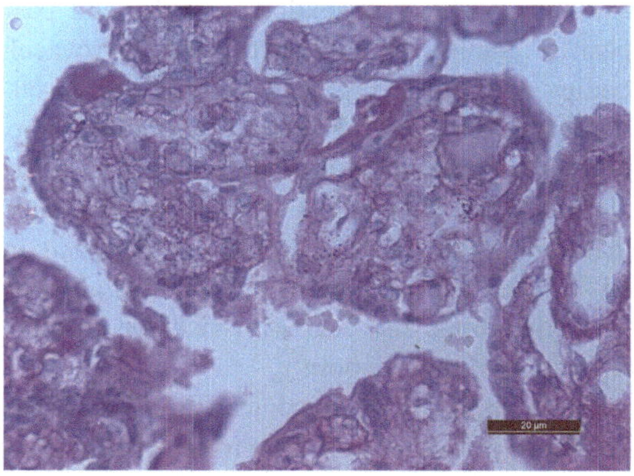

Fig. 5.18 Numerous extra- and intracellular PAS-positive inclusions in stem villi ×600

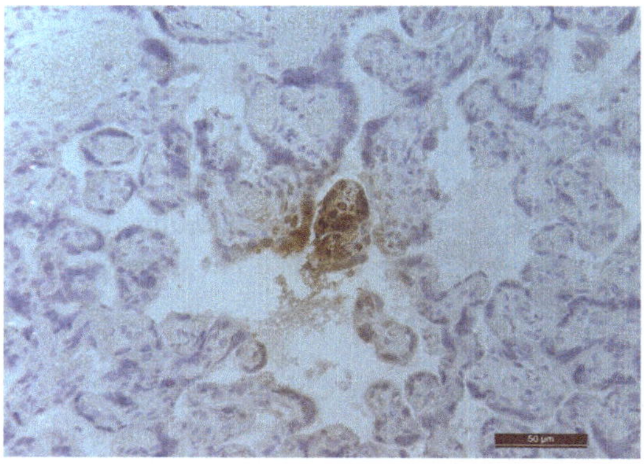

Fig. 5.19 Chlamydia trachomatis antigen in villi. IHC ×300

infected with chlamydia at birth. In the clinic of intrauterine chlamydia, it is customary to distinguish between local (conjunctivitis, gastroenterocolitis, atypical pneumonia) and generalized forms of infection. Among the most important manifestations of generalized chlamydia infection, it is customary to consider meningoencephalitis, cardiomyopathy, pneumonia, gastroenteritis, hepatitis, lymphadenitis, often complicated by the development of DIC syndrome. In a significant part of those infected (up to 22%), there are no clinical manifestations of the disease in the early neonatal period, an exacerbation of the process may occur throughout the first year of life and even later, when the connection with intrauterine infection may no longer be traced.

It is important to note that currently urogenital and intrauterine chlamydia are a very important problem in animal husbandry, especially in cattle. In bulls with genital chlamydia, testicular lesions are noted in 100% of cases (in the form of small-focal necrotic or chronic sclerosing orchitis), in 96%—serous fibrinous or adhesive periorchitis, in 86%—catarrhal urethritis, less often chronic postitis, prostatitis, vesiculitis, cuperitis. In calves with intrauterine chlamydia, gastroenteritis, pneumonia, hepatitis, nephritis, meningoencephalitis, polyarthritis and bursitis are considered the most typical. In many localizations, the intracellular location of the pathogen is shown.

Morphological changes in fetal/child tissues are either not discussed at all in the literature or are regarded as non-specific and described in total without taking into account possible mixed infectious lesions. This served as the basis for the analysis of their own materials. The diagnosis of chlamydia was made on the basis of a comparison of clinical and anamnestic data (in many cases, the detection of chlamydia in the mother), the results of morphological examination and IF detection of extracellular and intracellular forms of chlamydia in smears from different organs (commercial diagnostic serums for *C. trachomatis* from various domestic and foreign manufacturers were used). The results of the analysis for one of the perinatal departments of St. Petersburg for the year are presented.

As a result of the analysis of 104 autopsies of fetuses and newborns, intrauterine chlamydia as the main disease was the direct cause of death in 12 cases.

At the same time, chlamydial placentitis was accompanied by chronic placental insufficiency, manifested by the presence of a large amount of fibrinoid, thrombosis of the intervillous space, pseudoinfarcts, massive calcification, sclerosis, etc. Intrauterine chlamydia was generalized with damage to a number of internal organs and the central nervous system, which indicates a transplacental infection. In acute placental insufficiency or in chronic compensated placental insufficiency with acute decompensation, accompanied by disorders of uteroplacental circulation, which led to intranatal fetal hypoxia, the manifestations of chlamydia were minimal, mainly with damage to the respiratory organs, which indicates an ascending path of infection. At the same time, the immediate cause of fetal death was asphyxia or related complications. Comparison of the results of histological and immunofluorescence studies in the diagnosis of chlamydia in fetuses and in the study of afterbirth (showed a coincidence of the results obtained using these methods.

The morphological manifestations of chlamydia consisted in a peculiar transformation of cells of various origins, which were determined in various affected organs (Figs. 5.20 and 5.21). The cytoplasm increased quite significantly in size, becoming finely vacuolized. At the same time, fine grain was determined in it, which is better fixed when stained with azur-eosin and Schiff reagent.

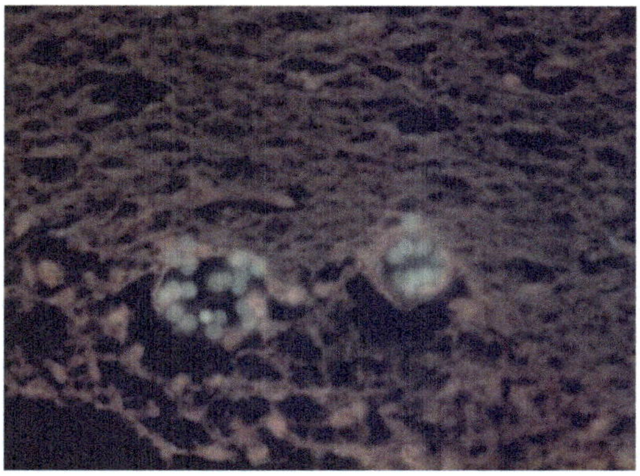

Fig. 5.20 Chlamydia antigen in lung. Immufluorescent microscopy ×600

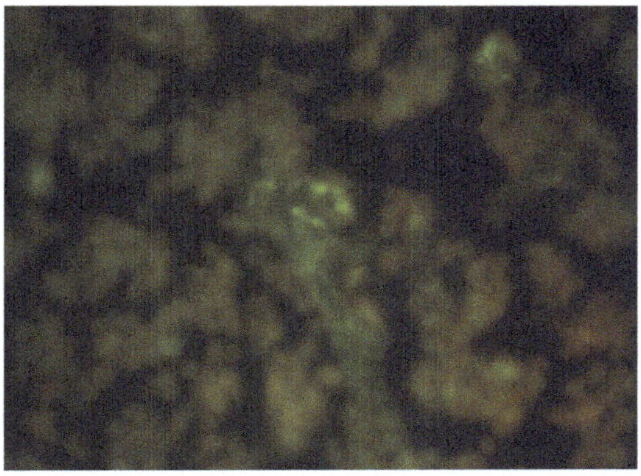

Fig. 5.21 Chlamydia antigen in heart. Immufluorescent microscopy ×600

Currently, the attention of a number of researchers from the Ural region of Russia [90] in intrauterine chlamydia is attracted by damage to the brain, especially the soft meninges. The authors describe the appearance of peculiar granulomas in them, which are already determined macroscopically on the convexital surface of the brain in the form of "cotton-like" formations (Fig. 5.22). Using EM, chlamydia was determined inside the cells of these granulomas (Fig. 5.23). In our material, such pronounced changes in soft meninges are not naturally determined. When studying them purposefully in observations with verified generalized intrauterine chlamydia, we noted a slight increase in the number of fibroblasts in all observations, in about half of the cases with the formation of granuloma-like structures around the vessels. It can be assumed that these differences in soft meninges lesions may be related to differences in the properties of strains circulating in different regions.

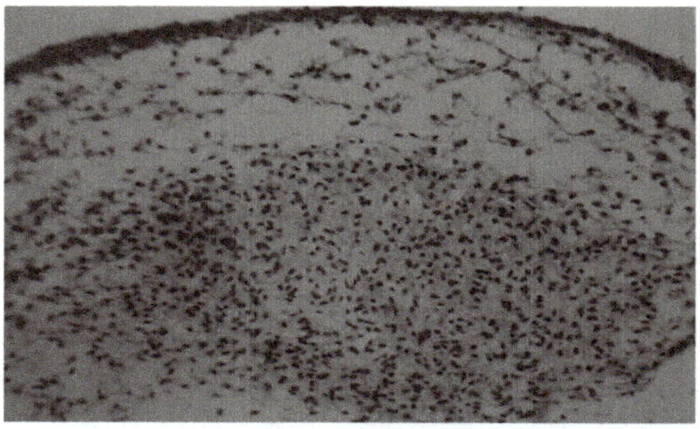

Fig. 5.22 Granuloma in soft meninges in intrauterine chlamydiosis. H-E. ×50. (Courtesy of S.A. Zworygin)

In another study, we analyzed 49 sectional observations of children who died from intrauterine infections. To confirm the chlamydial etiology of the process, the serum Chlamonoscrin-2 was used, designed to detect Cl. Trachomatis. The drug is monoclonal mouse antibodies specific to protein antigens of all Cl. trachomatis serotypes.

As a result of the study, a positive result was obtained in 21 cases (42.9%).

In this group, there were 13 girls (61.9%) and 8 boys (38.1%), full-term children—14 (66.7%), premature babies—7 (33.3%). Stillbirth was noted in 12 cases (57.1%): 6 children died antenatally, 6 intranatally, 7 children (33.3%) died in the first 3 days. Two children (9.6%) died at an older age of 24 days and 1.5 months.

In cases of stillbirth (group 1) and death of children in the first 3 days (group 2), the main diagnosis was intrauterine infection (IUI) with damage to various organs. In children who died at a later date (group 3), IUI appeared as a background pathology, and the main cause of death in the first case was generalized viral infection, in the second—acute intestinal infection (E. coli O-26).

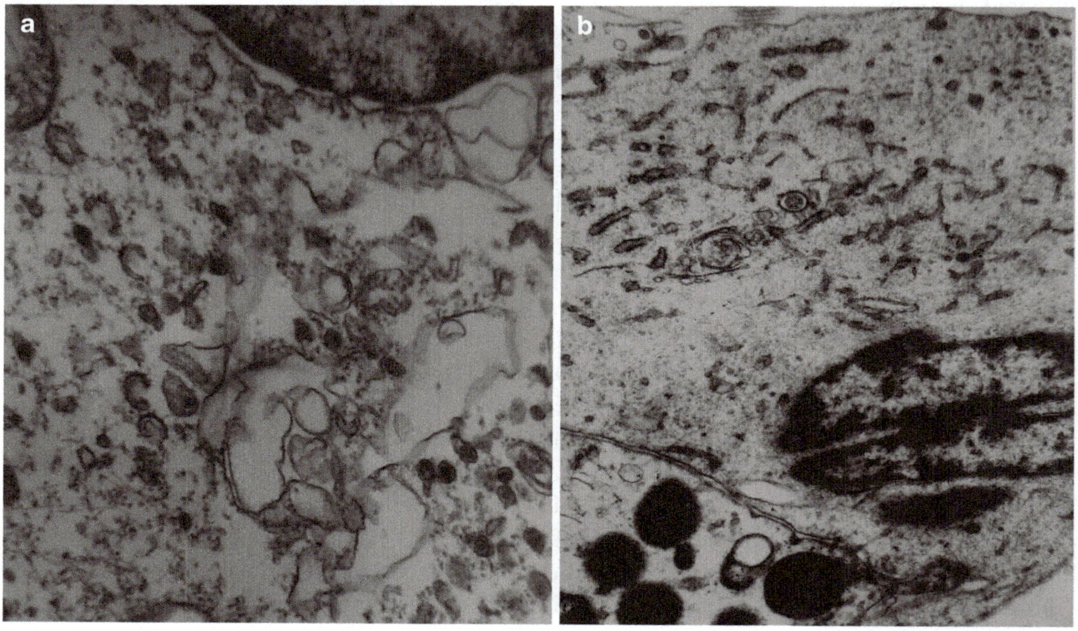

Fig. 5.23 Electron microscopy of brain meninges. (**a**) Hydropic necrosis of meningocyte with vacuole formation. In cytoplasm numerous elementary and intermediate bodies of Chlamydia. ×12,000. (**b**) Active fibroblast contacts with meningocyte containing reticular bodies of Chlamydia. ×14,000. (Courtesy of S.A. Zworygin)

In all cases, dewaxed preparations of the kidneys, liver, lung, brain, and heart were studied when using the luminescent microscopy.

In the first group of children, glow was observed in the kidneys in all cases, and only in the kidneys in three observations. Other combinations of organs in which luminescence were noted in this group: kidney + liver—in 5 observations; kidney + lung + liver—3; kidney + lung—1 observation.

In the second group of children, the following combinations of luminescence in organs were observed: isolated in the kidneys—in 3 observations; kidney + liver—2; kidney + lung—2 observations.

In the third group, in 1 case, the glow was only in the kidneys, in the second, the combination of kidney + lung + liver.

Thus, in all cases, the glow was observed in the kidneys, both in isolation and in various combinations with the liver and lungs. In none of the cases was there a positive reaction in the heart and brain tissue.

Pronounced morphological changes in IUI were noted:

In the first group (stillborn children), various combinations of organ lesions: liver + brain tissue—7 observations; liver + soft meninges (sm)—1 observation; liver + brain tissue +SM—2; liver + brain tissue + lungs 1; liver + brain tissue + sm + lungs—1 observation. Thus, in this group, liver damage was noted in all cases, in most cases the brain was involved in the process.

In the second group, the following combinations of organ lesions were noted: lung + liver + brain tissue + soft meninges (mmo)—1 observation; lungs + liver + brain tissue—3; lungs + brain tissue—2; liver + brain tissue—1 observation. These data show that in the second group, the structure of organ damage is somewhat different. In 6 of their 7 cases, the involvement of lungs in the process is also noted. This allows you to think about different ways of infection.

In the third group, in both cases, the liver and brain tissue were involved in the process.

During pathomorphological examination, pronounced circulatory disorders (fullness, hemorrhages), distelectases, desquamation of the epithelium, mainly macrophage infiltration with a small admixture of eosinophilic leukocytes, leukocytes and lymphocytes were noted in the lungs. In the liver—fullness, dystrophic changes, discomplexation of hepatic beams, abundance of islands of extramedular hematopoiesis, lympho-macrophage infiltration around the triads and along the portal tracts, small-scale hepatocyte dystrophy, in cases of still-birth, hepatocytes with cytoplasm emptying were noted. From the side of the brain tissue—edema phenomena, dystrophic cell changes, fullness of blood, perivascular inflammatory infiltrates and foci of gliosis. It should be noted that in the kidneys, where the glow was noted in all cases, there were no specific morphological changes characterizing the infectious process. The processes of circulatory disorders and dystrophic changes in the epithelium of the tubules were determined. There were no significant differences in the morphological picture in all groups.

Nearby typical histological changes Chlamydia antigen was detected in several organs by IHC (Figs. 5.24, 5.25 and 5.26).

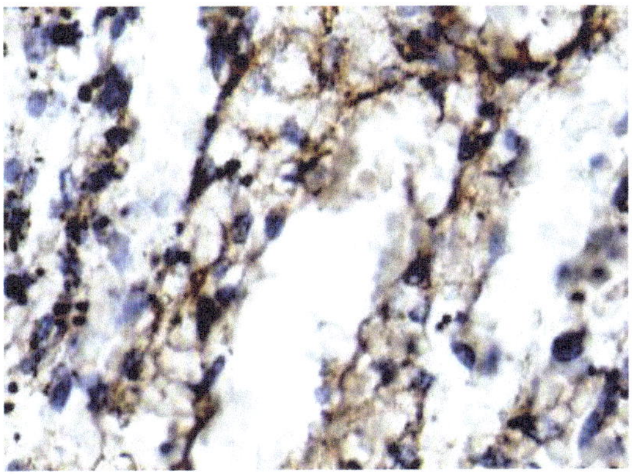

Fig. 5.24 Chlamydia trachomatis antigen in kidney. IHC. ×600

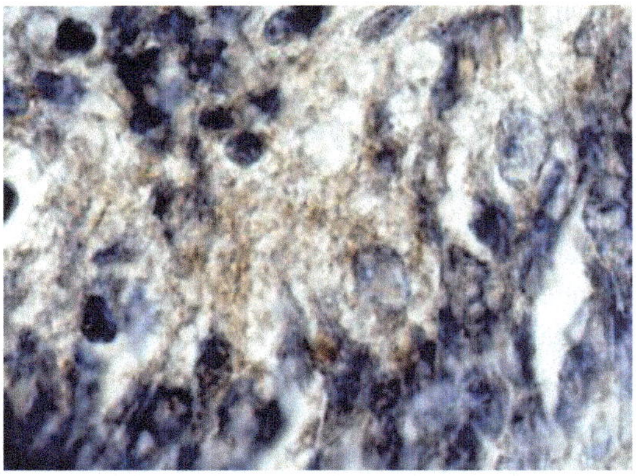

Fig. 5.25 Chlamydia trachomatis antigen in ependyma cells. IHC. ×600

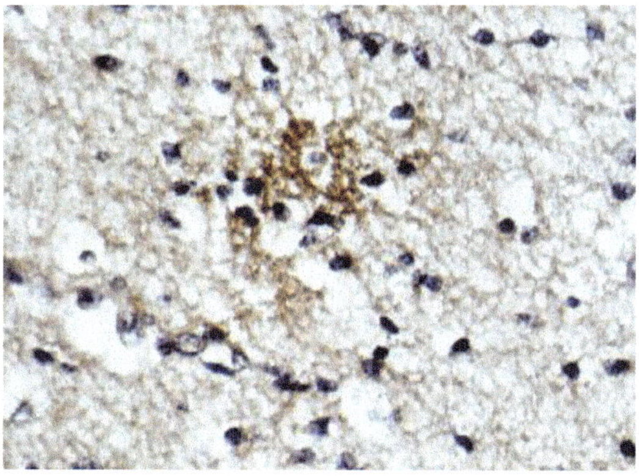

Fig. 5.26 Chlamydia trachomatis antigen in brain matter. IHC ×400

5.3 Conclusions

- Intrauterine infection with chlamydia can be both intranatal and antenatal
- Intrauterine chlamydia occurs as a generalized infection with damage to two or more organs The data provided by our studies of various years, performed using various methods, clearly indicate a significant frequency of perinatal chlamydia. Various pathogens from this group can play an etiological role in the development of pathology of pregnancy, fetus, newborn, and older children. The nature of the clinical manifestations of the disease can vary significantly from practically asymptomatic to fatal, with the most characteristic being the chronic course. Morphological changes in chlamydia of different localizations are similar, although they are little known and can be used in diagnosis. Many issues related to the epidemiology, pathogenesis and morphological manifestations of chlamydial infections need further study.
- Given the positive reaction in the kidneys with immunofluorescence and the absence of pronounced morphological manifestations, it can be assumed that the kidney is the organ where the pathogen can persist.

References

1. Megli CJ, Coyne CB. Infections at the maternal-fetal interface: an overview of pathogenesis and defense. Nat Rev Microbiol. 2021;20:67–82. https://doi.org/10.1038/s41579-021-00610-y.
2. Delorme-Axford E, Sadovsky Y, Coyne CB. The placenta as a barrier to viral infections. Annu Rev Virol. 2014;1(1):133–46. https://doi.org/10.1146/annurev-virology-031413-085524.
3. Silasi M, Cardenas I, Kwon JY, et al. Viral infections during pregnancy. Am J Reprod Immunol. 2015;73(3):199–213. https://doi.org/10.1111/aji.12355.
4. Yong HEJ, Chan SY, Chakraborty A, et al. Significance of the placental barrier in antenatal viral infections. Biochim Biophys Acta Mol basis Dis. 2021;1867(12):166244. https://doi.org/10.1016/j.bbadis.2021.166244.
5. Deblonde J, Claeys P, Temmerman M. Antenatal HIV screening in Europe: a review of policies. Eur J Public Health. 2007;17(5):414–8.
6. Schäfer A, Jovaisas E, Stauber M, Löwenthal D, Koch MA. Proof of diaplacental transmission of HTLV III/LAV before the 20th week of pregnancy. Geburtshilfe Frauenheilkd. 1986;46(2):88–9.
7. Soilleux EJ, Coleman N. Transplacental transmission of HIV: a potential role for HIV binding lectins. Int J Biochem Cell Biol. 2003;35(3):283–7.
8. Weber DJ, Redfield RR, Lemon SM. Acquired immunodeficiency syndrome: epidemiology and significance for the obstetrician and gynecologist. Am J Obstet Gynecol. 1986;155(2):235–40.
9. Drake AL, John-Stewart GC, Wald A, Mbori-Ngacha DA, et al. Herpes simplex virus type 2 and risk of intrapartum human immunodeficiency virus transmission. Obstet Gynecol. 2007; 109(2 Pt 1):403–9.
10. Thea DM, Steketee RW, Pliner V, Bornschlegel K, et al. The effect of maternal viral load on the risk of perinatal transmission of HIV–1. New York City Perinatal HIV Transmission Collaborative Study Group. AIDS. 1997;11(4):437–44.

11. Tubiana R, Le Chenadec J, Rouzioux C, Mandelbrot L, et al. Factors associated with mother–to–child transmission of HIV–1 despite a maternal viral load <500 copies/ml at delivery: a case–control study nested in the French perinatal cohort (EPF–ANRS CO1). Clin Infect Dis. 2010;50(4):585–96.
12. Douglas G, Fazely CF, Hu JJ. Transmission of HIV to the placenta, fetus and mother and implications of gametic infection. J Reprod Immunol. 1998;41(1–2):321–9.
13. Newman L, Rowley J, Vander Hoorn S, Wijesooriya NS, Unemo M, Low N, et al. Global estimates of the prevalence and incidence of four curable sexually transmitted infections in 2012 based on systematic review and global reporting. PLoS One. 2015;10(12):e0143304.
14. Tsai CA, Hung JK, Weiser DS. Is food insecurity associated with HIV risk? Cross-sectional evidence from sexually active women in Brazil. PLoS Med. 2012;9(4):e1001203.
15. Vogenthaler SN, Kushel BM, Craig H, Frongillo AE Jr, Riley DE, Bangsberg RD, et al. Food insecurity and risky sexual behaviours among homeless and marginally housed HIV-infected individuals in San Francisco. AIDS Behav. 2013;17(5):1688–93.
16. Mitjà O, Padovese V, Folch C, Rossoni I, Marks M, et al. Epidemiology and determinants of reemerging bacterial sexually transmitted infections (STIs) and emerging STIs in Europe. Lancet Reg Health Eur. 2023;34:100742. https://doi.org/10.1016/j.lanepe.2023.100742.
17. Gottlieb SL, Low N, Newman LM, Bolan G, Kamb M, Broute N. Toward global prevention of sexually transmitted infections (STIs): the need for STI vaccines. Vaccine. 2014;34:1527–35.
18. Adler M, Cowan F, French P, Mitchell L, Richens J. ABC of sexually transmitted infections. 5th ed. BMJ Publishing Group, London; 2004.
19. Anderson I, Robson B, Connolly M, Al-Yaman F, Bjertness E, King A, et al. Indigenous and tribal peoples' health (The Lancet–Lowitja Institute Global Collaboration): a population study. Lancet [Internet]. 2016 [cited 2021 Sep 21];388:131–57. https://www.thelancet.com/journals/lancet/article/PIIS0140-6736(16)00345-7/fulltext.
20. Gracey M, King M. Indigenous health part 1: determinants and disease patterns. Lancet [Internet]. 2009 [cited 2020 Dec 22];374:65–75. https://linkinghub.elsevier.com/retrieve/pii/S0140673609609144.
21. Minichiello V, Rahman S, Hussain R. Epidemiology of sexually transmitted infections in global indigenous populations: data availability and gaps. Int J STD AIDS [Internet]. 2013 [cited 2021 Sep 21];24:759–68. http://journals.sagepub.com/doi/10.1177/0956462413481526.
22. Centers for Disease Control and Prevention. Congenital syphilis (Treponema pallidum) 2015 case definition. 2015 [cited 2020 Jan 28]. https://ndc.services.cdc.gov/case-definitions/congenital-syphilis-2015/.
23. WHO | The global elimination of congenital syphilis: rationale and strategy for action [Internet]. World Health Organization [cited 2021 Sep 21]. https://www.who.int/publications/i/item/9789241595858.
24. Korenromp EL, Rowley J, Alonso M, Mello MB, Wijesooriya NS, Mahiané SG, et al. Global burden of maternal and congenital syphilis and associated adverse birth outcomes—estimates for 2016 and progress since 2012. PLoS One [Internet]. 2019 [cited 2021 Sep 21];14:e0211720. https://journals.plos.org/plosone/article?id=10.1371/journal.pone.0211720.
25. Russell NK, Nazar K, del Pino S, Gonzalez MA, Bermúdez XPD, Ravasi G. HIV, syphilis, and viral hepatitis among Latin American Indigenous Peoples and Afro-descendants: a systematic review. Rev Panam Salud Publica [Internet]. 2019 [cited 2021 Sep 21];43:1–13. http://iris.paho.org/xmlui/handle/123456789/49727.
26. Benirschke K, Burton GJ, Baergen RN. Pathology of the human placenta. 6th ed. Berlin: Springer; 2012, 941p.
27. Greco MA, Wieczorek R, Sachdev R, Kaplan C, Nuovo GJ, Demopoulos RI. Phenotype of villous stromal cells in placentas with cytomegalovirus, syphilis, and nonspecific villitis. Am J Pathol. 1992;141(4):835–42.
28. Qureshi F, Jacques SM, Reyes MP. Placental histopathology in syphilis. Hum Pathol. 1993;24(7):779–84.
29. Folgosa E, Osman NB, Gonzalez C, Hägerstrand I, Bergström S, Ljungh A. Syphilis seroprevalence among pregnant women and its role as a risk factor for stillbirth in Maputo, Mozambique. Genitourin Med. 1996;72(5):339–42. https://doi.org/10.1136/sti.72.5.339.
30. Guarner J, Southwick K, Greer P, et al. Testing umbilical cords for funisitis due to Treponema pallidum infection, Bolivia. Emerg Infect Dis. 2000;6(5):487–92.
31. Zinserling VA, Melnikova VF. Perinatal infections: questions of pathogenesis, morphological diagnostics and clinic–pathological correlations. Practical manual. SPb: Elbi–SPb. 2002, 352p. (In Russian).
32. Zinserling AV, Zinserling VA. Modern infections. Pathological anatomy and pathogenesis issues. Guide. 2nd ed., supplemented and revised. SPb: Sotis; 2002, 352p. (in Russian).
33. Kolobov AV, Karev VE, Vorobtsova IN, Orel VI. Intrauterine infections with nonimmune hydrops fetalis. J Infectologii. 2013;5(2):109–12. (In Russian).
34. Thomas J, Govender N, McCarthy KM, Erasmus LK, Doyle TJ, et al. Outbreak of listeriosis in South Africa associated with processed meat. N Engl J Med. 2020;382:632–43.
35. Al-Tawfiq JA. Listeria monocytogenes bacteremia in a twin pregnancy with differential outcome: fetus papyraceus and a full-term delivery. J Microbiol Immunol Infect. 2008;41:433–6.
36. Chan BT, Hohmann E, Barshak MB, Pukkila-Worley R. Treatment of listeriosis in first trimester of pregnancy. Emerg Infect Dis. 2013;19:839–41.

37. Chan LM, Lin HH, Hsiao SM. Successful treatment of maternal Listeria monocytogenes bacteremia in the first trimester of pregnancy: a case report and literature review. Taiwan J Obstet Gynecol. 2018;57:462–3.
38. Mylonakis E, Paliou M, Hohmann EL, Calderwood SB, Wing EJ. Listeriosis during pregnancy: a case series and review of 222 cases. Medicine (Baltimore). 2002;81:260–9.
39. Megli CJ, Coyne CB. Infections at the maternal–fetal interface: an overview of pathogenesis and defence. Nat Rev Microbiol. 2022;20(2):67–82. https://doi.org/10.1038/s41579-021-00610-y.
40. Megli C, Morosky S, Rajasundaram D, Coyne CB. Inflammasome signaling in human placental trophoblasts regulates immune defense against Listeria monocytogenes infection. J Exp Med. 2021;218:e20200649.
41. Robbins JR, Skrzypczynska KM, Zeldovich VB, Kapidzic M, Bakardjiev AI. Placental syncytiotrophoblast constitutes a major barrier to vertical transmission of Listeria monocytogenes. PLoS Pathog. 2010;6:e1000732.
42. Phelps CC, et al. Relative roles of Listeriolysin O, InlA, and InlB in Listeria monocytogenes uptake by host cells. Infect Immun. 2018;86:e00555–18.
43. Disson O, et al. Conjugated action of two species-specific invasion proteins for fetoplacental listeriosis. Nature. 2008;455:1114–8.
44. Holch A, Ingmer H, Licht TR, Gram L. Listeria monocytogenes strains encoding premature stop codons in inlA invade mice and Guinea pig fetuses in orally dosed dams. J Med Microbiol. 2013;62:1799–806.
45. Lecuit M, Nelson DM, Smith SD, Khun H, Huerre M, Vacher-Lavenu M-C, Gordon JI, Cossart P. Targeting and crossing of the human maternofetal barrier by Listeria monocytogenes: role of internalin interaction with trophoblast E-cadherin. Proc Natl Acad Sci USA. 2004;101:6152–7.
46. Bakardjiev AI, Theriot JA, Portnoy DA. Listeria monocytogenes traffics from maternal organs to the placenta and back. PLoS Pathog. 2006;2:623–31.
47. Faralla C, et al. Listeria monocytogenes InlP interacts with afadin and facilitates basement membrane crossing. PLoS Pathog. 2018;14:e1007094.
48. Parkash V, et al. Immunohistochemical detection of Listeria antigens in the placenta in perinatal listeriosis. Int J Gynecol Pathol. 1998;17:343–50.
49. Azari S, Johnson LJ, Webb A, Kozlowski SM, Zhang X, Rood K, Amer A, Seveau S. Hofbauer cells spread Listeria monocytogenes among placental cells and undergo pro-inflammatory reprogramming while retaining production of tolerogenic factors. mBio. 2021;12(4):e01849–21. https://doi.org/10.1128/mBio.01849-21. Published online 2021 Aug 17.
50. Dramsi S, Lévi S, Triller A, Cossart P. Entry of Listeria monocytogenes into neurons occurs by cell-to-cell spread: an in vitro study. Infect Immun. 1998;66:4461–8. https://doi.org/10.1128/IAI.66.9.4461-4468.1998.
51. Drevets DA, Sawyer RT, Potter TA, Campbell PA. Listeria monocytogenes infects human endothelial cells by two distinct mechanisms. Infect Immun. 1995;63:4268–76. https://doi.org/10.1128/iai.63.11.4268-4276.1995.
52. Le Monnier A, Autret N, Join-Lambert OF, Jaubert F, Charbit A, Berche P, Kayal S. ActA is required for crossing of the fetoplacental barrier by Listeria monocytogenes. Infect Immun. 2007;75:950–7. https://doi.org/10.1128/IAI.01570-06.
53. Portnoy DA, Auerbuch V, Glomski IJ. The cell biology of Listeria monocytogenes infection: the intersection of bacterial pathogenesis and cell-mediated immunity. J Cell Biol. 2002;158:409–14. https://doi.org/10.1083/jcb.200205009.
54. Kim J-S, Romero R, Kim MR, Kim YM, Friel L, Espinoza J, Kim CJ. Involvement of Hofbauer cells and maternal T cells in villitis of unknown aetiology. Histopathology. 2008;52:457–64. https://doi.org/10.1111/j.1365-2559.2008.02964.x.
55. Kim CJ, Romero R, Chaemsaithong P, Kim J-S. Chronic inflammation of the placenta: definition, classification, pathogenesis, and clinical significance. Am J Obstet Gynecol. 2015;213:S53–69. https://doi.org/10.1016/j.ajog.2015.08.041.
56. Kim MJ, Romero R, Kim CJ, Tarca AL, Chhauy S, LaJeunesse C, Lee D-C, Draghici S, Gotsch F, Kusanovic JP, Hassan SS, Kim J-S. Villitis of unknown etiology is associated with a distinct pattern of chemokine up-regulation in the feto-maternal and placental compartments: implications for conjoint maternal allograft rejection and maternal anti-fetal graft-versus-host disease. J Immunol. 2009;182:3919–27. https://doi.org/10.4049/jimmunol.0803834.
57. Charlier C, Disson O, Lecuit M. Maternal-neonatal listeriosis. Virulence. 2020;11:391–7. https://doi.org/10.1080/21505594.2020.1759287.
58. Becroft DM, Farmer K, Seddon RJ, Sowden R, Stewart JH, Vines A, et al. Epidemic listeriosis in the newborn. Br Med J. 1971;3:747–51.
59. Lamont RF, Sobel J, Mazaki-Tovi S, Kusanovic JP, Vaisbuch E, Kim SK, Uldbjerg N, Romero R. Listeriosis in human pregnancy: a systematic review. J Perinat Med. 2011;39(3):227–36.
60. Lennon D, Lewis B, Mantell C, Becroft D, Dove B, Farmer K, et al. Epidemic perinatal listeriosis. Pediatr Infect Dis. 1984;3:30–4.
61. Badri MS, Zawaneh S, Cruz AC, Mantilla G, Baer H, Spellacy WN, et al. Rectal colonization with group B streptococcus: relation to vaginal colonization of pregnant women. J Infect Dis. 1977;135:308–12.
62. Boyer KM, Gadzala CA, Burd LI, Fisher DE, Paton JB, Gotoff SP. Selective intrapartum chemoprophylaxis of neonatal group B streptococcal early-onset disease. I. Epidemiologic rationale. J Infect Dis. 1983;148:795–801.
63. Dillon HC Jr, Gray E, Pass MA, Gray BM. Anorectal and vaginal carriage of group B streptococci during pregnancy. J Infect Dis. 1982;145:794–9.

64. Halliday HL, Hirata T. Perinatal listeriosis-a review of twelve patients. Am J Obstet Gynecol. 1979;133:405–10.
65. Mazor M, Froimovich M, Lazer S, Maymon E, Glezerman M. Listeria monocytogenes. The role of transabdominal amniocentesis in febrile patients with preterm labor. Arch Gynecol Obstet. 1992;252:109–12.
66. Facinelli B, Varaldo PE, Casolari C, Fabio U. Cross-infection with Listeria monocytogenes confirmed by DNA fingerprinting. Lancet. 1988;2:1247–8.
67. Gunther G, Philipson A. Oral trimethoprim as follow-up treatment of meningitis caused by Listeria monocytogenes. Rev Infect Dis. 1988;10:53–5.
68. Posfay-Barbe KM, Wald ER. Listeriosis. Pediatr Rev. 2004;25:151–9.
69. Quarles JM Jr, Pittman B. Unsuccessful attempt to detect Listeria monocytogenes in healthy pregnant women. J Bacteriol. 1966;91:2112–3.
70. Schuchat A, Lizano C, Broome CV, Swaminathan B, Kim C, Winn K. Outbreak of neonatal listeriosis associated with mineral oil. Pediatr Infect Dis J. 1991;10:183–9.
71. Centers for Disease Control and Prevention. Preliminary FoodNet data on the incidence of infection with pathogens transmitted commonly through food—10 states, 2007. MMWR Morb Mortal Wkly Rep. 2008;57:366–70.
72. Albritton WL, Cochi SL, Feeley JC. Overview of neonatal listeriosis. Clin Invest Med. 1984;7:311–4.
73. Linnan MJ, Mascola L, Lou XD, Goulet V, May S, Salminen C, et al. Epidemic listeriosis associated with Mexican-style cheese. N Engl J Med. 1988;319:823–8.
74. McLauchlin J. Human listeriosis in Britain, 1967–85, a summary of 722 cases. 1. Listeriosis during pregnancy and in the newborn. Epidemiol Infect. 1990;104:181–9.
75. Schwarze R, Bauermeister CD, Ortel S, Wichmann G. Perinatal listeriosis in Dresden 1981–1986: clinical and microbiological findings in 18 cases. Infection. 1989;17:131–8.
76. Tessier F, Bouillie J, Daguet GL, Barrat J. [Listeriosis in obstetrical environment. Report on 10-year experience in a maternity hospital in Paris]. J Gynecol Obstet Biol Reprod (Paris). 1986;15:305–13.
77. Braden CR. Listeriosis. Pediatr Infect Dis J. 2003;22:745–6.
78. Henle A. Pseudotuberkulose bei neugebornen Zwillingen. Gottingen: Arb Pathol Inst; 1893.
79. Kelly CS, Gibson JL. Listeriosis as a cause of fetal wastage. Obstet Gynecol. 1972;40:91–7.
80. Albritton WL, Wiggins GL, Feeley JC. Neonatal listeriosis: distribution of serotypes in relation to age at onset of disease. J Pediatr. 1976;88:481–3.
81. Skidmore AG. Listeriosis at Vancouver General Hospital, 1965–79. Can Med Assoc J. 1981;125:1217–21.
82. Cruikshank DP, Warenski JC. First-trimester maternal Listeria monocytogenes sepsis and chorioamnionitis with normal neonatal outcome. Obstet Gynecol. 1989;73:469–71.
83. Fleming AD, Ehrlich DW, Miller NA, Monif GR. Successful treatment of maternal septicemia due to Listeria monocytogenes at 26 weeks' gestation. Obstet Gynecol. 1985;66:52S–3S.
84. Zervoudakis IA, Cederqvist LL. Effect of Listeria monocytogenes septicemia during pregnancy on the offspring. Am J Obstet Gynecol. 1977;129:465–7.
85. Miele K, Morris SB, Tepper NK. Tuberculosis in pregnancy. Obstet Gynecol. 2020;135(6):1444–53. https://doi.org/10.1097/AOG.0000000000003890.
86. Sugarman J, Colvin C, Moran AC, Oxlade O. Tuberculosis in pregnancy: an estimate of the global burden of disease. Lancet Glob Health. 2014;2:e710–6.
87. Centers for Disease Control and Prevention. Who should be tested. https://www.cdc.gov/tb/topic/testing/whobetested.htm. Accessed 17 Feb 2020.
88. Sobhy S, Babiker Z, Zamora J, Khan KS, Kunst H. Maternal and perinatal mortality and morbidity associated with tuberculosis during pregnancy and the postpartum period: a systematic review and meta-analysis. Br J Obstet Gynaecol. 2017;124:727–33.
89. Bogdanova EV, Kiselevich OK, Yusubova AN, Sevostyanova TA, Shirshov IV, Klimov GV, Zyuzya YR, Alvarez Figeroa MV, Dolgova EA. Inborne tuberculosis. Tuberculez i bolezni legkih. 2012;90(1):54–8. (In Russian).
90. Samokhin PA, Erman BA, Tulakina LG, et al. Morphological characteristics of intrauterine chlamydiosis and its clinic-anatomical characteristics. Arkh Patol. 1997;59(5):27–31. (In Russian).

6 Transplacental Transmission Infections: Viral Infections

6.1 Infections Due to Hepatitis B and C Viruses

Nearby lesions of liver in adult and children due to postnatal infections inborn hepatitis have been described centuries ago. Nowadays, it is admitted that the main role in their etiology play viruses B and C. Certain similarities in epidemiology, clinical features, and morphological picture allows to analyze them in the same chapter.

Hepatitis B virus (HBV) is a partially double-stranded DNA virus, belonging to the Hepadnaviridae family of viruses, whereas hepatitis C virus (HCV) is a small, enveloped, positive-sense single-stranded RNA virus of the Flaviviridae family [1, 2]. They are both transmitted via blood or non-sterile needle use (through drug injections, tattoos or medical procedures) or via sexual contacts [3]. The global prevalence of hepatitis C virus (HCV) infection is 2–3%, with 130–170 million HCV-positive people—most of them chronically infected [4]. The epidemiology of HCV is varies among countries and the reported prevalence of HCV in pregnant women has not been extensively studied, due to the lack of preventative screening of infection and the lack of preventative measures of mother-to-child transmission.

Hepatitis B surface antigen (HBsAg) is a particle produced in excess during the life cycle of the virus: HBsAg is the first detectable viral antigen to appear during infection but could also be later found, whereas core antigen (HBcAg) and envelope antigen (HBeAg) are indicators of active viral replication [3]. Anti-HBs antibodies can be detected after seroconversion or after a successful anti-HBV immunization, while HBV-DNA is a feasible marker to monitor viral load [5]. The maternal HBV carrier status prevalence varied from regions. It has been reported that 5.5–15.5% of pregnant women are infected with HBV in Asia and Africa, and 1.6–2.6% in the USA and Europe [6–9]. Pregnancy complications related to HBV infection if any are minimal. Prior evidence demonstrates that HBV infection during pregnancy contributes to an increased risk of adverse obstetrical (gestational diabetes, antepartum hemorrhage, preeclampsia) and neonatal outcomes, including preterm birth (relative risk (RR) = 1.24, 95% CI: 1.19–1.33), miscarriage (adjusted OR (aOR) = 1.71, 95% CI: 1.23–2.38), macrosomia (aOR = 1.68, 95% CI: 1.19–2.37), and low-birth weight (RR = 1.26, 95% CI: 1.05–1.51) [10–13]. The risk of mother-to-child transmission (MTCT) of HBV is dependent on the timing of exposure: in the case of a HBV-infected mother in the third trimester, the risk is higher and vertical transmission will occur in 80–90% [14].

The pathogenesis of HCV infection during pregnancy remains poorly understood. During pregnancy, the maternal immune system must at the same time develop tolerance to paternal alloantigens to prevent maternal immune aggression

V. Zinserling et al., *Placentitis and Perinatal Infections*,
https://doi.org/10.1007/978-3-031-80553-0_6

against the fetus and maintain active immunity against HCV to protect both mother and fetus from infection [15]. Moreover, it is important to define the effect of pregnancy on HCV and vice versa. Finally, understanding the transmission of HCV to infants and the risk factors correlated with transmission will provide information for counseling and management of HCV infection during puerperium. There is no unfavorable effect of HCV on pregnancy [16].

In a population-based cohort study using Washington state birth records from 2003 to 2005, including 506 HCV-positive mothers, 2022 randomly selected HCV-negative mothers, and 1439 drug-using HCV-negative mothers, it was shown that infants born to HCV-positive women were more likely to have low-birth weight, be small for gestational age, be admitted to the intensive care unit, or require assisted ventilation [17].

In a more recent study using birth certificate records of 1,670,369 pregnancies, it was found that women with HCV were more likely to have infants born preterm, with low-birth weight and congenital anomalies [18]. However, that study had several limitations, in particular, its retrospective design and the lack of association with several variables, such as use of tobacco, alcohol, or drugs. Indeed, there is no explanation for prematurity and low-birth weight in HCV-negative mothers, although increased cytotoxicity of placental natural killer T cells could be hypothesized possibility [19].

The presence of HCV-RNA indicates active infection: the risk of vertical transmission of HCV is reduced in women with an undetectable HCV-RNA, although an intermittent viral load could lead to vertical transmission [20]. Approximately, HCV infection occurs in 6–11% of infants born to HCV-infected mothers [2, 21]. Co-infection with HIV increases the rate of mother-to-child transmission up to 19.4% [22]. The weighted rate of transmission is 8.6% in mothers who are anti-HCV positive and injecting drug users, compared with 3.4% in anti-HCV-positive mothers without known injecting drug use. A meta-analysis including 2382 infants estimated that the risk of HCV vertical transmission was 2.82 from anti-HCV+/HIV+ co-infected mothers compared with anti-HCV+/HIV− mothers [23]. Vertical transmission of HIV and HCV separately is most likely from HIV/HCV-co-infected mothers; however, transmission of both infections is less frequent [24].

Numerous risk factors for vertical transmission have been studied. In general, high viral load defined as at least 2.5×10^6 viral RNA copies/mL, HIV co-infection, and invasive procedures are the most important factors [25]. In general, maternal peripheral blood mononuclear cell infection by HCV, membrane rupture >6 h before delivery, and procedures exposing the infant to maternal blood infected with HCV during vaginal delivery are associated with an increased risk of transmission [26]. Abnormal ALT levels in mothers in the year before pregnancy may reflect a more severe liver disease and may help in identifying mothers with an increased risk of vertical transmission [27]. Finally, a Japanese study suggested that maternal liver dysfunction, large blood loss at delivery, and vaginal delivery were potential novel risk factors for mother-to-child transmission of HCV [28].

Transplacental leakage (related to immature placenta or uterine contractions), placental infection, and infected maternal peripheral blood mononuclear cells (that turn out to be HBV carriers from mother to fetus) have been described as potential mechanisms for HBV intrauterine transmission, considering that only HBeAg is small enough to cross placenta [29]. During pregnancy, significant changes in maternal immune system usually occur to avoid rejection of the semiallogenic fetus. The natural course of HBV infection is influenced by a depressed maternal cell-mediated immunity, that could stimulate MTCT and the development of an immune-tolerant HBV infection in the fetus [30, 31]. Although acute HBV infection during pregnancy is not associated with increased fetal mortality or teratogenicity, a higher risk of gestational diabetes, postpartum hemorrhage, preterm birth, and low-birth weights was reported among complications of HBV-infected pregnant women [5, 30, 32]. Vertically, HBV-infected infants are usually asymptomatic and anicteric, but they are likely to have a chronic infection afterwards in 90% of cases [33].

As in other viral infections, human trophoblast cells express cellular receptors (Occludin, Claudin-1, and low-density lipoproteins receptor) that HCV use to enter into host cells. This leads to a strong antiviral response that alters innate immunity at the maternal–fetal interface. Furthermore, immunologic changes trigger apoptotic pathway in extra-villous trophoblast cells, altering placental morphology: this probably plays a key role in pregnancy-related complications: women with HCV infection are more likely to have stillborn infants or infants born preterm, with low-birth weight or birth defects [18, 34, 35].

When the placenta is damaged by hepatitis B, C viruses, microscopically, according to our data, the most characteristic are endovasculitis of small and large vessels of the decidua and stem villi. The nuclei of endothelial cells increase in size, become juicy and polymorphic (Fig. 6.1). Particularly characteristic are changes in the nuclei of decidual cells, in which, against a hyperchromic background, round pale oxyphilic inclusions of various sizes, characteristic of viral hepatitis, are detected (in 87%). Often (62%) large multinucleated decidual cells are identified [36].

In an IHC study, hepatitis B (usually when the mother has HBeAg in her blood) and hepatitis C antigens are detected primarily in the stroma and on the surface of stem (53%) and terminal (15.4%) villi and decidual cells (34.6%) (Figs. 6.2 and 6.3) [36].

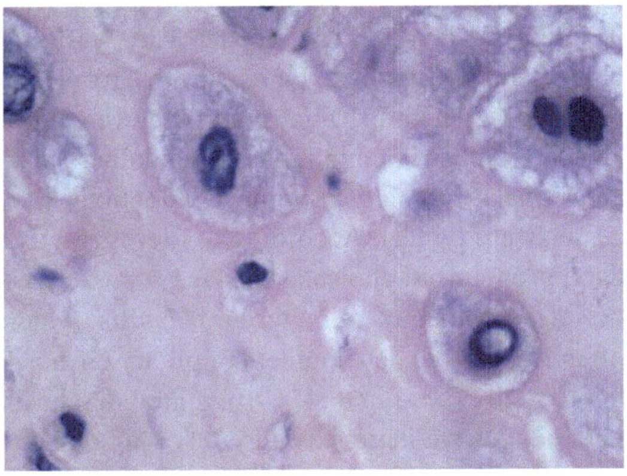

Fig. 6.1 Hepatitis B virus deciduitis. Note large pale intranuclear inclusion, H&E, ×1000

On our material, it is possible to identify four main variants of liver changes:

1. The most common are minimal or moderate changes characterized by increased extramedullary hematopoiesis, dystrophic changes in the cytoplasm of hepatocytes with moderately pronounced nuclear polymorphism, occasionally individual inclusions, not significantly pronounced inflammatory changes in the walls of the liver veins;
2. Giant cell hepatitis, characterized by the appearance of multinucleated cells several times larger than an ordinary hematocyte in the form of process-like symplastic structures, sometimes with a two-row chain of nuclei (Fig. 6.4). Focal nuclear polymorphism with indistinctly pronounced small light inclusions may be observed. Their cytoplasm, as in other less modified hepatocytes, contains numerous inclusions, glycogen, and small grains of bile pigments. In addition, there is a discomplexation of hepatic beams, phlebitis of the hepatic veins, cholestasis, proliferation of cholangioles with lymphohistiocyte infiltration around them. There is also a pronounced collagenization of the stroma to varying degrees. Such changes, often referred to by the term "giant cell hepatitis of newborns," can also be observed in older children. Isolated observations of this kind suggest that the mechanism of formation of giant cells in these observations is associated with an immune defect—Bruton syndrome).
3. Hepatitis resembling acute viral hepatitis in adults. According to the materials of Leningrad/ St. Petersburg, such observations are extremely rare, often in the form of a sectional find (Fig. 6.5).
4. Hepatitis, resembling chronic viral hepatitis in adults, with discomplexation of the hepatic beams and pronounced fibrosis around the central veins and in the area of the portal tracts, similar to adult hepatitis. This form of hepatitis in newborns has been rarely observed in recent years.

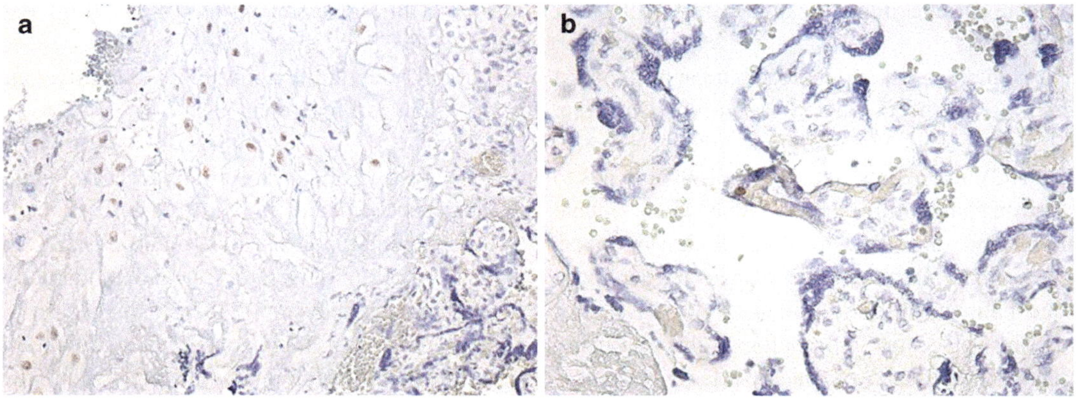

Fig. 6.2 Expression of HBcAg in decidua cells (**a**) and endotheliocytes (**b**), IHC, ×200

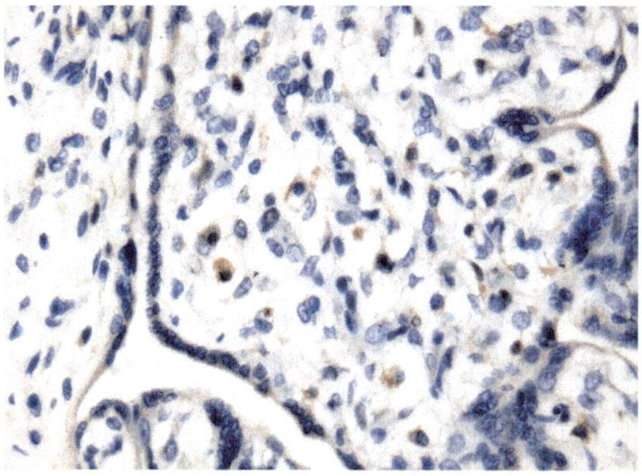

Fig. 6.3 Expression of HC-Ag in Hofbauer cells, IHC, ×400

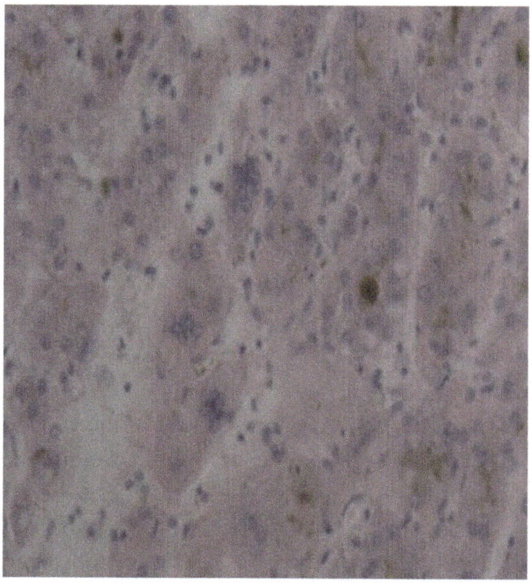

Fig. 6.4 Chronic intrauterine giant cell hepatitis with cholestasis/ H-E ×600

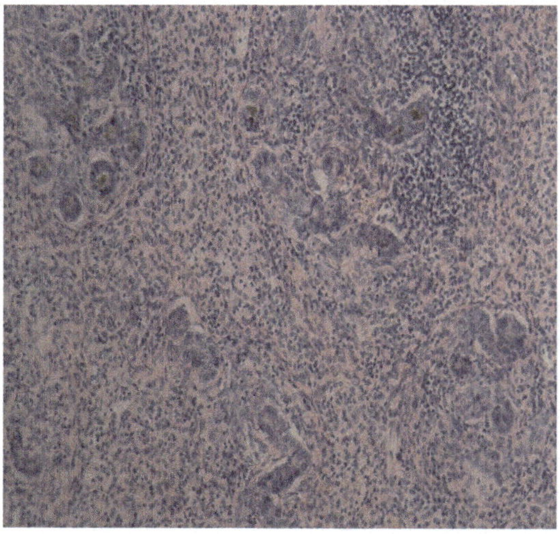

Fig. 6.5 Chronic intrauterine hepatitis B. H-E. ×400

Analysis of the course of intrauterine viral hepatitis) indicates a significant variety of its clinical manifestations. Jaundice, hepatosplenomegaly, and hemorrhagic syndrome were very characteristic. Combinations with other both ante- and postnatally developed infectious processes were typical. According to morphological data, pronounced cholestasis is very characteristic of the course of intrauterine hepatitis, which often leads to the development of biliary cirrhosis in the future (see Fig. 6.4). Differential diagnosis with congestive jaundice caused by various non-inflammatory factors should be carried out with particular care.

The detection of the morphological picture of cirrhosis in the liver of a newborn child forces, taking into account the literature data, to carry out differential diagnosis with a number of rare hereditary pathologies: Wilson-Konovalov disease, galactosemia, insufficiency of antitrypsin, etc., in which the development of intrauterine cirrhosis with tissue restructuring is considered characteristic Having no own experience in studying biochemically and genetically confirmed diseases of this group, we can only note the need for careful exclusion with appropriate diagnoses of intrauterine viral hepatitis according to all histological and laboratory criteria.

6.2 Human Immunodeficiency Virus Infection

Infection due to Human immunodeficiency virus (HIV) has been intensively studied by different specialists in the recent decades. Notable that in numerous researches presenting pathological changes main attention was drawn to secondary infections and tumors, while changes related to direct virus effect were revealed seldom. Our scientific school described in different organs cell changes we consider as typical for HIV lesion.

Transplacental transmission of human immunodeficiency virus ranks second in terms of the “efficiency” of infection (the first place is the transfusion of infected blood) and can occur at any time, but more often in the last month of pregnancy. HIV enters the child with placental defects, leading to the penetration of the virus into the bloodstream of the fetus [37, 38]. The risk of intrauterine transmission of HIV from mother to child depends on many factors. It is high during acute HIV infection and during maternal AIDS [39, 40]. The presence of HIV RNA in the mother’s blood at a concentration of more than 1000 copies/ml is associated with the risk of infection of the fetus. The main factors of intrauterine HIV infection are: high levels of HIV RNA in the mother’s blood on the eve of childbirth, lack of chemoprophylaxis during pregnancy, childbirth and in newborns, and evidence that pregnant women are drug users [41].

The possibility of infection of the fetus with a low viral load in the mother is associated with a number of factors—the presence of other infections in the woman, including sexually transmitted infections, poor maternal nutrition, smoking, injecting drug use [40, 42, 43]. In addition, inflammatory processes in the placenta play a role (acute chorioamnionitis, placentitis) [37]. Contact of the blood of an HIV-infected mother and the secretion of her birth canal with the skin and mucous membranes of the fetus at the time of delivery can also lead to infection of the child. Long anhydrous gap increases the risk of perinatal HIV transmission by two times [44, 45]. It is extremely significant that HIV-1 contamination of the amniotic fluid was not observed even in cases of HIV infection, accompanied by a high titer of the virus in the blood plasma. This is in contrast to the effective secretion of viral particles in breast milk, which determines the high importance of the lactation mechanism of HIV transmission [45, 46].

Infection of the placental tissue itself does not determine the penetration of viral particles to the fetus [47, 48]. It is assumed that the rate of progression of infection in infants depends on the subclass of the virus received from the mother. At the same time, infection with a strain of the virus with a high degree of replication and the formation of syncytium are associated with a high degree of probability of the rapid development of AIDS. First of all, the placenta is a physical barrier to the virus. Also, a number of studies have shown that the human placental trophoblast may not have HIV interaction factors or have a virus replication limiting factor, which prevents infection of these cells by HIV-1 [49]. For example, an obstacle to the penetration of HIV into the placenta is the syncytial nature of the trophoblast (syncytiotrophoblast) and the ability to synthesize nitric oxide and interferons [36]. The secretion of IL-2 and γ-interferon in the placental tissue with HIV infection is significantly reduced, and IL-4 and IL-1β is increased. In particular, in the villous chorion, inflammatory infiltrates are noted, represented by cells producing IL-2, IL-4 and IL-1β, and the secretion of the anti-inflammatory cytokine IL-4 predominates. Both in cases with uncomplicated pregnancy and with HIV infection, the content of IL-1β in the villous chorion was insignificant and the cause of impaired maturation of the villous chorion in defective differentiation of the villi [41].

CD14-expressing cells of the immune system play a role in HIV transmission. So, Marlin et al. [50] note the important role of macrophages and dendritic cells in the pathogenesis of HIV infection using the example of CD14+ cells of the decidua.

The similarity of the HIV antigen gp120 with the antigens of trophoblast cells was noted, as well as the possibility of direct transmission of HIV from infected lymphocytes to trophoblast cells by endocytosis. In experiments on cell cultures, the possibility of latent infection of placental cells of monocytic origin has been proven. At the same time, HIV replication is regulated by cytokines produced by the infected cells themselves [41].

Currently, there is convincing evidence that under conditions of adequate treatment of HIV-infected pregnant women, the risk of infection of the newborn, determined by PCR of peripheral blood, is minimal. At the same time, there are integrated forms of HIV, in which the virus is not detected in the peripheral blood. Cytomegalovirus infection of newborn children from women with HIV infection is observed more than ten times more often [41].

HIV infection in pregnant women in 84.5% of cases is combined with other genital infections [51–55]. In addition, herpesvirus infection is also characterized by association with other infectious agents—chlamydia, opportunistic bacteria [56]. At the same time, the threat of early miscarriage increases, in particular, when associated with chlamydial infection—1.7 times [57]. The frequency of preterm birth in HIV-infected pregnant women is 17.1%, and in cases of perinatal infection of the fetus increases to 43.9%.

Changes in the placenta and extraplacental membranes in HIV infection are detected primarily in the trophoblast, endotheliocytes of fetal vessels and cells of the stroma of the villi, which increase in size, mainly due to light, large nuclei with a part of an irregular shape [58–61]. Using the immunoperoxidase method, viral proteins were detected in Hofbauer cells. In other studies using immunohistochemistry and in situ hybridization, the possibility of detecting HIV in trophoblast cells, amniotic epithelium, lymphocytes, and decidual tissue has been proven [62, 63]. Also, in the villous chorion, vasculopathy occurs with the formation of fibrin thrombi, diffuse lymphoid infiltration and edema of the stroma of the villi [64]. There is a violation of the maturation of the villi, often with focal dissociation of their development. Groups of immature villi are determined, partly with clusters of Hofbauer cells in the edematous stroma. With HIV infection in all placentas, there are manifestations of chronic placental insufficiency with non-specific involutive changes expressed to varying degrees and acute circulatory disorders. In addition, Jauniaux et al. [59] noted in their 50 observations a significant decrease in the placental–fetal index. In a study by Vermaak et al. [65] also found a decrease in placental mass in HIV-infected pregnant women. These researchers also drew attention to the increase in the frequency of marginal infarcts in the placenta.

Also, with HIV infection in the placenta, there is a violation of collagen synthesis. Thus, type III collagen ("young collagen") is present in the terminal villi not only in the stroma, but also in the structure of the vasculosyncytial basement membrane, which leads to its thickening. In addition, increased collagen formation is also noted in the walls of the vessels of the stem and intermediate villi. An increased content of type I collagen is noted in the treated HIV infection, and in the absence of antiretroviral therapy, the optical density of this type of collagen corresponds to normal values. The optical density of type IV collagen is reduced in the placentas of HIV-infected women who did not receive antiretroviral therapy, and in the group treated with HIV infection, the content of type IV collagen in the vascular wall and in the composition of the vasculosyncytial basement membrane exceeds the standard values [41].

Placentas of HIV-infected pregnant women in the implementation of vertical transmission of HIV are characterized by a violation of the maturation of the villi with stromal fibrosis and perivillous fibrinoid deposits, which was regarded as a morphological substrate of chronic subcompensated placental insufficiency.

An in-depth study of 78 placentas with HIV infection in the mother received during term delivery from 2005 to 2011 was carried out in St. Petersburg.

The placentas of HIV-infected women are characterized by impaired maturation of villi with stroma fibrosis, the formation of fibrinoid and petrificates, which were the morphological substrate of chronic placental insufficiency with varying degrees of compensation. In our study, morphological signs of placental insufficiency were detected in 100.0% of cases, and in all cases, it was chronic subcompensated placental insufficiency.

Infection of the placenta and extraplacental membranes was noted in all cases, and inflammatory changes of bacterial etiology (chorioamnionitis, membranitis) amounted to 75.0%.

Viral lesions were represented by the action of the RNA virus and were manifested by giant cell metamorphosis of trophoblast cells and macrophages of the villus stroma, as well as infiltration of the placenta with immunocompetent cells.

Groups of immature villi with edematous stroma and large cells with light nuclei are determined. It is notable that similar changes were described by us in different tissues in HIV-virus infection. Numerous symplastic structures, as a rule, with large light nuclei were also determined in the decidual tissue. In all placentas, p24 expression was noted in trophoblast cells, villus stroma, and decidual cells during immunohistochemical studies. This protein is the main structural core protein of the HIV virion and allows you to verify HIV infection.

In our study, morphological signs of placental insufficiency were detected in 100.0% of cases, and in all cases, it was chronic subcompensated placental insufficiency.

Infection of the placenta and extraplacental membranes was noted in all cases, and inflammatory changes of bacterial etiology (chorioamnionitis, membranitis) amounted to 75.0%.

Viral lesions were represented by the action of the RNA virus and were manifested by giant cell metamorphosis of trophoblast cells and macrophages of the villus stroma as well as infiltration of the placenta with immunocompetent cells.

Groups of immature villi with edematous stroma and large cells with light nuclei are determined. It is notable that similar changes were described by us in different tissues in HIV-virus infection. Numerous symplastic structures, as a rule, with large light nuclei were also determined in the decidual tissue. In all placentas, p24 expression was noted in trophoblast cells, villus stroma, and decidual cells during immunohistochemical studies. This protein is the main structural core protein of the HIV virion and allows you to verify HIV infection.

In our study in the placentas with mother's HIV infection and the absence of vertical transmission of HIV, an increase in the expression of CD14 and a decrease in the expression of FasL were noted (Fig. 6.6a). In the placentas with mother's HIV infection and realized vertical transmission of HIV, an imbalance between pro- and anti-angiogenic factors due to increased expression of TGF-β1, Tsp-1, and decreased expression of CD14 and CD31 (Fig. 6.6b). This indicates a significant decrease in the number of Hoffbauer cells and reduction of blood vessels in cases with realized vertical transmission of HIV.

Children with congenital HIV infection are usually asymptomatic at birth: symptoms usually occur after 3 months and within 10 years, with lymphadenopathy, weight of loss, recurring infections, and a progressive developmental delay. Among the most typical pathological changes was encephalitis (Fig. 6.7).

Antigen p24 could be revealed in different organs, especially thymus (Fig. 6.8).

Case: Clinical and Morphological Observation of Newborn with Congenital HIV Infection

Child B. was born on April 10, 2010 from the sixth pregnancy of three premature births at a

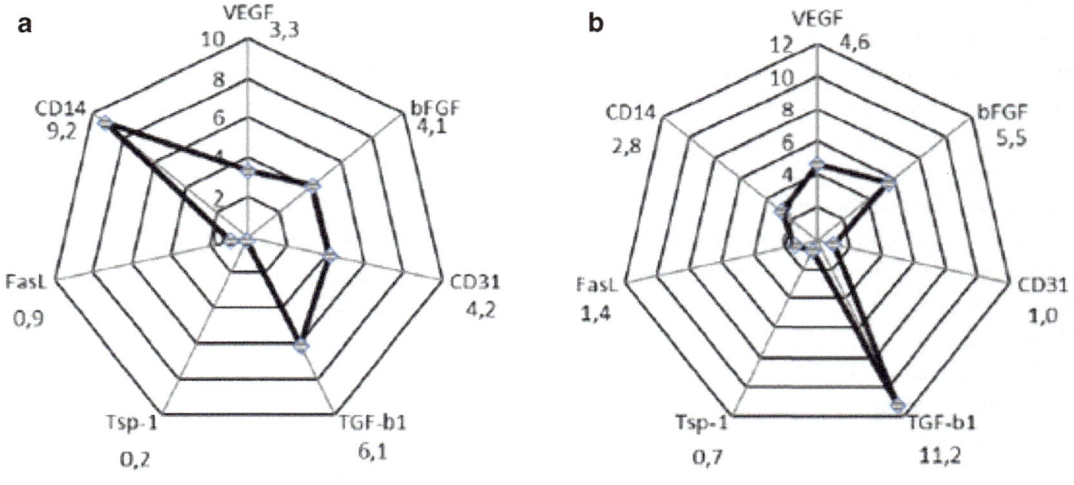

Fig. 6.6 Expression pro- and anti-angiogenic factors according to the relative area of expression (%) in placentas: (**a**) with HIV infection without vertical transmission of HIV; (**b**) with HIV infection during vertical transmission of HIV

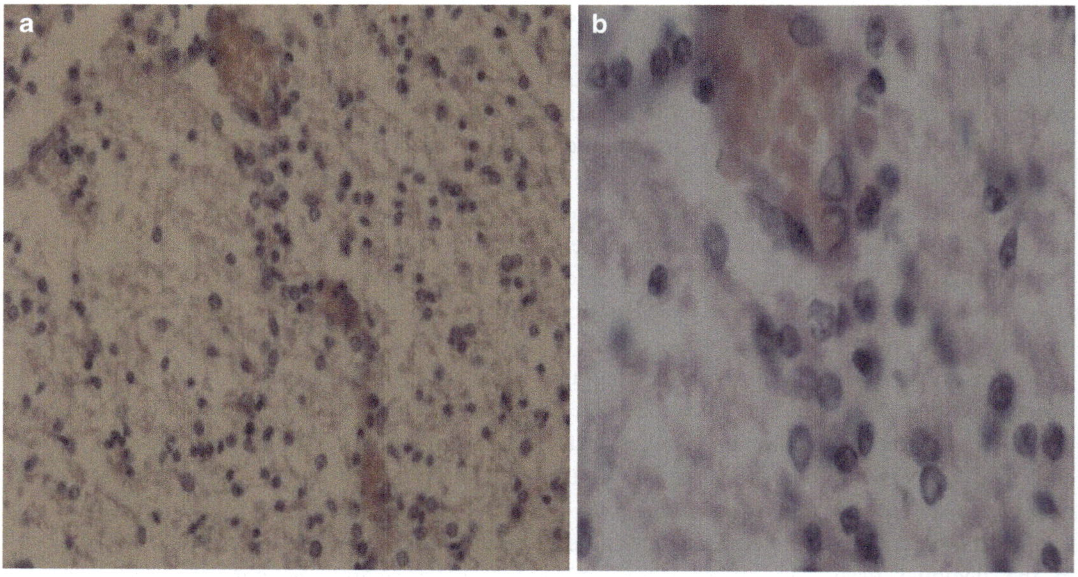

Fig. 6.7 Intrauterine HIV Encephalitis. H-E. (**a**) ×200, (**b**) ×600

gestational age of 35/36 weeks with a birth weight of 3180 g, a body length of 50 cm. According to the Apgar scale, the boy was rated at 6/7 points. The mother was registered at the AIDS center from 18 weeks of pregnancy, she was not observed in clinic. The mother did not receive specific antiretroviral therapy during pregnancy due to low adherence to observation. The maternal viral load before delivery was 88,300 copies/ml. Intrauterine infection was confirmed by a positive PCR result of HIV DNA from the newborn's blood, taken on the third day after birth. The infection of the child occurred due to the lack of antiretroviral prophylaxis during pregnancy against the background of a high viral load (88,300 copies/ml).

In the morphological study of the placenta and extraplacental membranes, signs of an infectious lesion of the afterbirth were noted—focal puru-

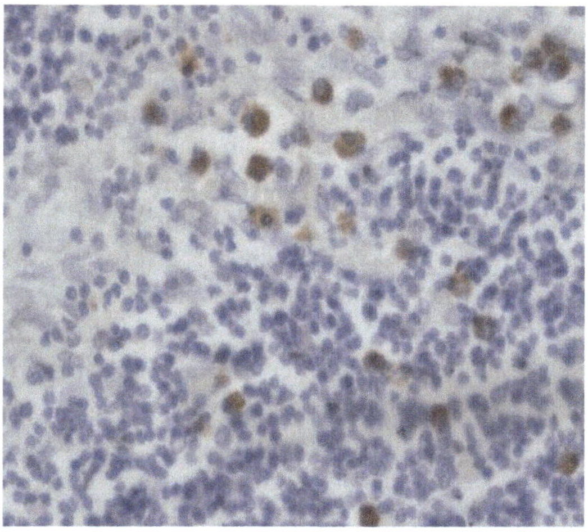

Fig. 6.8 P24 antigen in thymus of a newborn. IHC. ×600

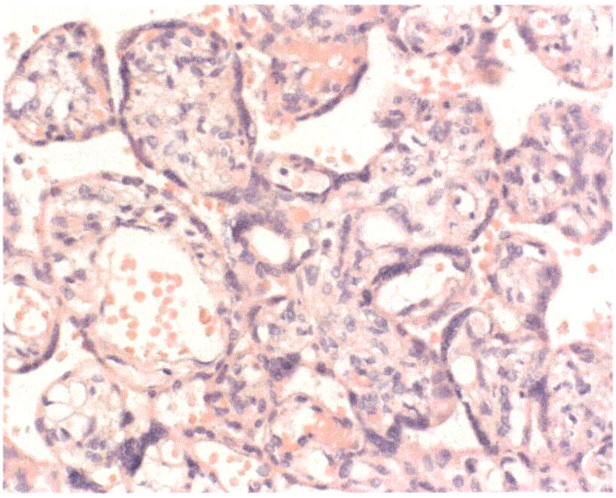

Fig. 6.9 Disturbance of branching and dissociated maturation of the villi with giant cell metamorphosis of the cells of the stroma of the villi; H&E, ×400

lent choriodeciduiitis and changes characteristic of HIV: giant cell metamorphosis of trophoblast cells and macrophages of the villus stroma, as well as infiltration of the placenta by immunocompetent cells (lymphocytes and macrophages) (Fig. 6.9). In addition, the revealed violation of the branching of the villous chorion with a predominance of intermediate villi, as well as the dissociated maturation of the villi, were regarded as a morphological substrate for chronic subcompensated placental insufficiency (Fig. 6.19). When conducting IHC with p24, an intense positive reaction was noted in placental macrophages (Fig. 6.10).

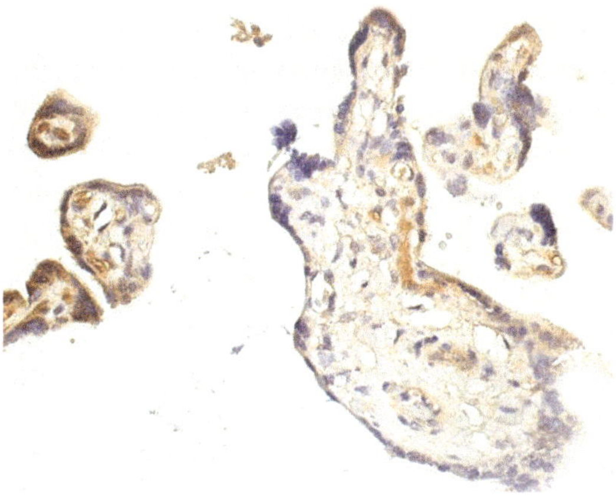

Fig. 6.10 Expression of p24 in placental macrophages and trophoblast, IHC, ×400

6.3 Herpes Simplex Virus Infection

Herpes simplex virus type 1 and 2 (HSV-1 and HSV-2) are DNA viruses belonging to Alphaherpesvirinae, a subfamily of the Herpesviridae family. Both of them, highly prevalent human pathogens, are transmitted across epithelial mucosal cells and skin discontinuations, migrate to the nerve tissues, and there are able to persist in a latent state. Although the viruses have different preferential site of infection, HSV-1 predominantly involving the trigeminal ganglia and HSV-2 the lumbosacral ganglia, both viruses are able to infect both the orofacial and the genital areas [66]. HSV infection is a sexually transmitted disease widely diffused in the world. Most cases of recurrent genital herpes are caused by HSV-2. It is estimated that in the USA almost 50 million people are infected with this type of virus [67]. Since the highest incidence of HSV infections involves women of reproductive age, the risk of maternal transmission to the fetus/neonate is a major health concern [66, 68–71]. The clinical condition characterized by acquisition of HSV-1 or HSV-2 without previous exposure to either virus or hence no preformed antibodies is referred to as "first-episode primary infection." In contrast, the clinical condition characterized by acquisition of HSV-2 in an individual with previous HSV-1 antibodies or vice versa is referred to as "first-episode nonprimary infection." In contrast, the term "reactivation" refers to the detection of HSV-1 in a patient who already has HSV-1 antibodies or of HSV-2 in a patient who already has HSV-2 antibodies [68, 72]. Recurrence and reactivation of the infection are much more frequent for HSV-2 than for HSV-1 genital infection and the prognosis and the type of counseling needed depend on the type of genital herpes (HSV-1 or HSV-2) causing the infection. It is therefore advisable that the clinical diagnosis of genital herpes is confirmed by type-specific laboratory tests and that positive subjects also be diagnosed for HIV, considering that genital HSV infection has long been identified as a risk factor in HIV acquisition, with a two- to threefold higher risk, also due to multiple sex partners. The biological basis of increased susceptibility is due to both increased ulceration and increased inflammation (with higher CD4+ cells) present in the skin and mucosa of HSV-2 infected individuals [73].

HSV infection process starts with virions binding to host cell surfaces, which triggers a cascade of multiple steps leading to penetration of viral genome into the nucleus, release of viral DNA for replication, capsid assembly, DNA packaging, envelopment via passage through the trans-Golgi network and host cell is destruction [72, 74].

Possible risk factors for HSV transmission to neonates include: (a) HSV serotype (HSV1 > HSV2); (b) type of maternal infection (recurrent HSV genital lesions are associated with lower risk for transmission to exposed neonates than primary HSV genital lesions; (c) maternal serostatus; (d) delivery mode (vaginal delivery > cesarean section); (e) prolonged duration of rupture of membranes; (f) impaired fetal cutaneous barriers (instrumentation-related) [68, 69, 72]. Timing of maternal infection is fundamental to establish: the risk for transmission of HSV infection to the neonate is high (30–50%) when women acquire genital HSV near the time of delivery and low (<1%) when women have prenatal history of recurrent HSV infections or who acquire genital HSV during the first half of pregnancy [75]. Vertical transmission of viral infection may occur during the intrauterine period (5%), in the peripartum period (85.9%) or postnatally (10%) [68, 69, 72]. HSV-1 prevalence was higher than HSV-2 at both maternal and fetal side of the placenta, evidencing how crossing of maternal-fetal interface is a common strategy used by HSV-1, whereas in the case of HSV-2 infection, the hematogenous route is more frequent [76].

Intrauterine HSV infection has been associated with encephalomalacia, hydrocephalus, calcifications, and microcephaly: HSV-infected neonates could display significant neurodevelopmental outcomes [77, 78].

With an exacerbation of HSV infection in pregnant women in the first trimester and an anti-HSV immunoglobulin titer of 1:6400-1:12,800, complications of pregnancy and childbirth, the incidence of newborns is higher than in pregnant women with an antibody titer of 1:1600-1:3200 [79]. In the presence of high titers of antibodies to HSV-1 and 2 (1:6400-1:12,800), the inferiority of the first and second wave of endovascular trophoblast migration is noted [80].

With herpes infection, there is often a discrepancy between the maturity of the placenta and the gestational age with a violation of the maturation of the villi, mainly in a dissociated type [79].

The herpes virus antigen leads to an increased release of proinflammatory interleukins into the peripheral blood of pregnant women. An increase in the ratios of pro- and anti-inflammatory cytokines at high titers of antibodies to HSV indicates a Th-1 pathway for the development of the mother's immunological response. Such a change in the cytokine status, which has a regulatory effect on the development of the immune response, is a reason to believe that the most sensitive to the effects of the herpes antigen was the suppressor activity of T-lymphocytes, the number of which was almost halved.

We succeeded to study 32 placentas with herpes simplex virus infection.

The villous chorion in all observations corresponded in terms of maturity to the term of full-term pregnancy. The morphological state was regarded as compensated on the basis of moderately pronounced compensatory-adaptive reactions due to active syncytial nodules and sufficient vascularization of the terminal villi. Involutive changes were mild and represented by minor deposits of fibrinoid and calcium in the peripheral parts of the placenta. Inflammatory changes in this subgroup were characterized by focal infiltrates predominantly in the basal lamina. Thus, a morphological study of the placentas of children with intrauterine herpesvirus infection revealed chronic subcompensated placental insufficiency in 53.1% of cases, chronic compensated placental insufficiency in 16.0%, and placental insufficiency was absent in another 30.9% of cases.

It has been established that full-term babies were born infected with HSV, regardless of the presence and severity of inflammatory changes in the placenta characteristic of herpes infection (placentitis, focal inflammatory changes or the absence of inflammatory changes). There was a diffuse mononuclear infiltration involving septa, stroma of the villi and extraplacental membranes, which was regarded as viral placentitis (Fig. 6.11). Changes characteristic of DNA-viral infections in the form of giant cell metamorphosis and hyperchromatosis of cell nuclei were noted in the extra-villous cytotrophoblast and villous syncytiotrophoblast, in the vascular endothelium and in the extraplacental membranes (Fig. 6.12). These changes were accompanied by small-lumpy disintegration of cell nuclei, primarily the basal lamina, with the formation of basophilic necrosis (Fig. 6.13). This indicates in favor of the hematogenous route of fetal herpesviruses infection. Pronounced compensatory-adaptive reactions (increased vascularization of the terminal villi, an increase in the number and size of syncytial nodes, thickening of vasculosyncytial membranes) prevented the implementation of the infectious process during fetal development [36].

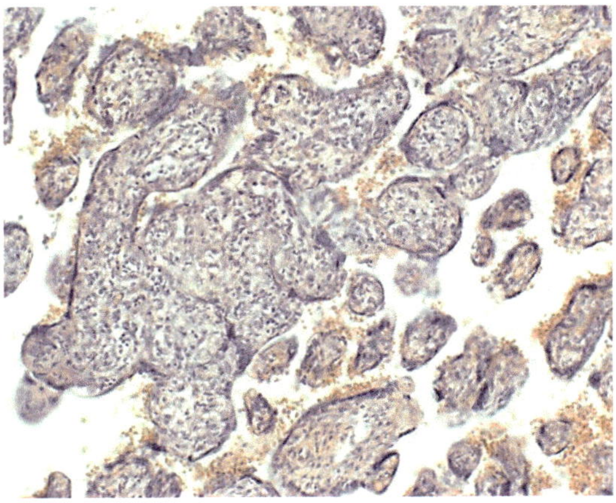

Fig. 6.11 Herpetic villitis, H-E, ×200

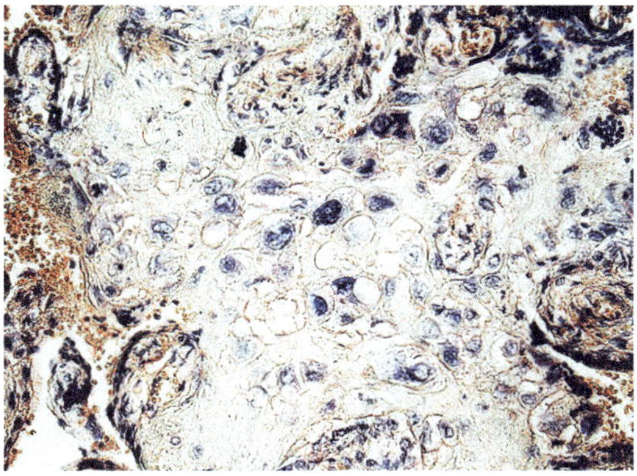

Fig. 6.12 Giant cell metamorphosis with hyperchromatosis of cell nuclei of peripheral cytotrophoblast, H-E, ×200

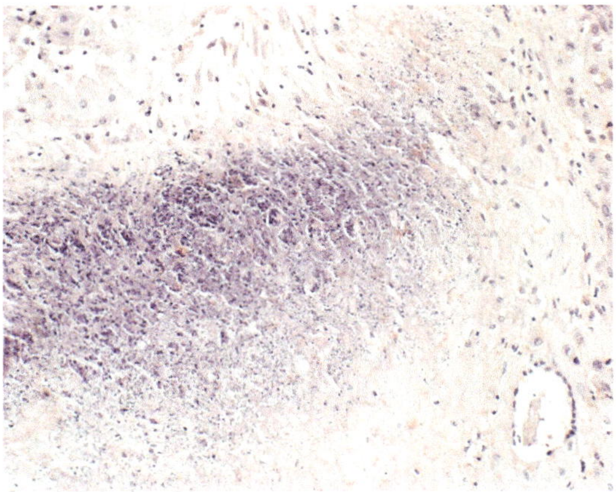

Fig. 6.13 Basophilic necrosis in the basal lamina in herpes infection, H-E, ×200

In an immunohistochemical study with antibodies to HSV types 1 and 2, a positive reaction was noted in infected cells (Fig. 6.14).

Different variants of the intrauterine herpes in the fetus (child) are possible—from severe antenatal herpes to the birth of a healthy child. Infection can also occur intranatally, especially in

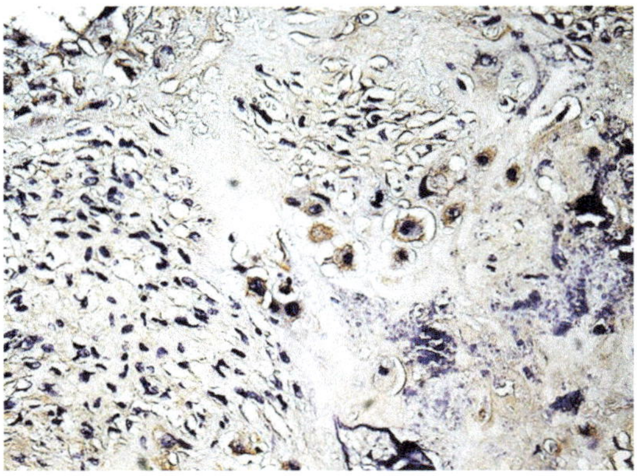

Fig. 6.14 Positive reaction with anti-HSV I/II antibodies, IHC study, ×200 the appointment of specific antiviral therapy. (Published with permission from Ref [17], an open access article distributed under the terms and conditions of the Creative Commons Attribution (CC BY) license)

the presence of genital herpes in the mother. There is an increase in spontaneous abortions and premature births against the background of herpes in the mother. The most likely way of infection with the development of severe forms of the disease with damage to the skin, conjunctiva of the eye, as well as the mucous membranes of the genitals is contact when the child passes through the infected birth canal of the mother. At the same time, it should be noted that 70% of mothers whose children were born with disseminated intrauterine germ had no signs of genital lesion during childbirth. Along with this, postnatal infection of the newborn is also possible.

In fact, the frequency of neonatal herpes remains unclear, the figures given vary significantly even in those countries where laboratory tests are conducted to search for this disease. The frequency of neonatal herpes varies between 1:5000 and 1:7500 births. The mortality rates of children in this age period are very high: without treatment from 18% (local form with skin and mucous membrane damage) to 90% (disseminated form); when treated with acyclovir, the mortality rate from the disseminated form decreases to 57%.

It should be noted that under seemingly equal conditions, lesions of the organs of a newborn can differ dramatically. Presents the results of a triplet examination. The first child developed severe skin herpes 5 h after birth, followed by meningoencephalitis. The second child had acute chorioretinitis. The third child had no clinical manifestations of herpes, however, at the age of 3.5 months, he died suddenly in the presence of a respiratory infection.

A particularly severe course with the highest degree of generalization is noted by clinicians in the second half of the first week of life. Among the clinical manifestations of the disease, fever or hypothermia, jaundice, drowsiness, vomiting, nausea, cyanosis, and rapidly developing acute circulatory insufficiency are indicated. The spleen and liver, as a rule, are enlarged. Dense yellowish mucus may accumulate in the larynx. Increased bleeding is associated with thrombocytopenia, liver failure, and DIC. In the final stage of the disease, shock and polio-induced insufficiency are described. The disease proceeds extremely unfavorably and usually ends fatally at 2–3 weeks. At this time, hemorrhagic syndrome may occur.

It is currently customary in the clinic to give especially great importance to CNS lesions. Using neurosonography, it was found that clinical variants of herpetic lesions may include panencephalitis with an outcome of multicystic encephalitis; periventricular encephalitis with the formation of cystic forms of periventricular leukomalacia; as well as intraventricular and periventricular hemorrhages. It should be noted that in the fatally terminated observations, a good correlation of the results of lifetime and postmortem studies was noted. Vegetative state, severe forms of cerebral palsy, oligophrenia, optic nerve atrophy, sensorineural hearing loss, mental development disorders, hydrocephalus are described as neurological consequences of such lesions. At the same time, it is noted that focal cortical-subcortical encephalitis, meningitis, ventriculitis, and choroiditis of herpetic etiology, diagnosed and treated in the neonatal period, are currently a manageable pathology with relatively favorable neurological outcomes.

Despite dozens of descriptions of fatal intrauterine herpes, they do not provide any detailed information about the pathological anatomy of this disease. Most often, only necrotic foci in different organs are described with the presence of enlarged cells with large nuclei containing intracellular inclusions around them. The most common reports are of intracranial calcifications, microcephaly, microophthalmia, retinal dysplasia, widespread necrosis of brain tissue leading to hydrocephalus and liver necrosis. In addition, there is information about possible skin lesions, short fingers and persistence of the arterial (Botall's) duct. Sometimes, there are not only single-core, but also multinucleated cells. Among the affected organs, changes in the liver, adrenal glands, lungs, brain, esophagus, tongue, large intestine, as well as spleen, lymph nodes, stomach, bone marrow, conjunctiva, pharynx, and heart are described.

The most complete information on the results of an EM study of the lungs of newborns who died of a herpetic infection is provided by Shabunina. As with other infections, type 2 alveolocytes, where virus reproduction was intensive, were subject to the greatest destructive changes. In the expanded cisterns of the endoplasmic network, the authors found a large number of nucleocapsids of the herpes simplex virus, around which numerous lysosomes were localized. In these cells, the cytoplasmic membrane was indistinct, its ruptures and the release of organelles into the light of the alveoli were noted in places. The mitochondria looked swollen, hypertrophied, with ruptured cysts and impaired membrane double-contour. The expansion of tubules and cisterns of the endoplasmic reticulum was noted. Cytoplasm in the places of virus reproduction acquired an osmiophilic appearance.The number of viral particles detected in different cells of the alveolar epithelium was different. Thus, single virions with a supercapsid shell were found in some cells. In others, the nucleocapsides were arranged in groups of 2–8 or more, surrounded by a membrane. Changes also occurred in the nuclei of cells. Chromatin was located unevenly in them: either along the edge of the nuclear membrane or in the form of lumpy clusters in the nucleoplasm. Changes in capillaries were expressed in swelling of endothelial cells, their enlightenment, and thinning of the basal membrane.

Once we had the opportunity to examine of the autopsy material out using different techniques (light microscopy, IF-examination of scraped smears from the affected organs, serological examination of the blood of the deceased, sometimes in combination with the same blood tests of his parents) [36]. The frequency of detection of herpes in deceased children turns out to be very significant. In our material, the disease was caused by HSV-1 and HSV-2 with the predominance of the latter. The structural changes revealed in the organs in herpes caused by HSV-1 and HSV-2 were practically indistinguishable from each other.

In the acute period of the disease, single-type changes in cells of predominantly epithelial origin are found in many organs. They are characterized by an increase in the size of the affected cells and their nuclei, fragmentation of chromatin, the marginal location of its lumps in the nucleus, the enlightenment of the central part of the nucleus with the presence of a large basophilic or eosinophilic inclusion, as well as a fine-grained cell degradation (probably apoptosis). With the most pronounced alterative changes, the death of individual cells or their groups with the formation of foci of necrosis is noted. As a rule, there is no cellular inflammatory reaction around the sites of alteration. In addition, blood circulation disorders and some other non-specific changes are detected. With a longer duration of the disease, the phenomena of regeneration and organization of exudate are observed.

Lesions in intrauterine herpes are localized in the same organs as in other intrauterine infections. They are most often detected in the liver, where acute hepatitis occurs with giant cell metamorphosis of both hepatocytes and Kupffer cells.

Macroscopically, the liver is slightly enlarged, flabby, mottled in the section, with the presence of small, sometimes merging grayish-yellow foci. Spot hemorrhages are often detected under the capsule. The possibility of developing necrotic focal or diffuse hepatitis has been described by many authors. On microscopic examination, the most typical are intracellular inclusions in hepatocytes in a state of hydropic dystrophy, mainly along the edges of necrotic foci. These inclusions can vary quite significantly both in size and color intensity. It seems to us that initially they have a distinct matte appearance associated with active replication of the virus. Later, the inclusion becomes darker, is intensely stained with hematoxylin, and sharply separates from other parts of the nucleus. Small oxyphilic inclusions can also be detected in the cytoplasm of infected cells. In the later stages, karyorexis is determined. Exudative reaction may be practically not expressed. An increase in extramedullary hematopoiesis is naturally determined. We also often observed lung damage—focal pneumonia. In the early stages of the disease, lumen of the alveoli contains liquid, small clusters of mononuclears and exfoliated, enlarged alveolocytes with a metamorphosis characteristic of herpes. An admixture of erythrocytes to the exudate is possible, and areas of alveolar decline are noted. With the greatest severity of the lesion, pronounced alterative changes occur with the formation of fields of coagulation necrosis of the lung tissue.

The brain is often affected. Morphological examination in the early stages of brain damage against the background of generalized herpes reveals swelling of individual neurons and glial cells, in the nuclei of which large basophilic inclusions are detected (Fig. 6.15). Hyperchromatosis of nuclei with fragmentation and marginal location of nuclear matter is often seen. In addition, signs of subependimar gliosis of varying severity are found. Macroscopically, such a brain is moderately flabby.

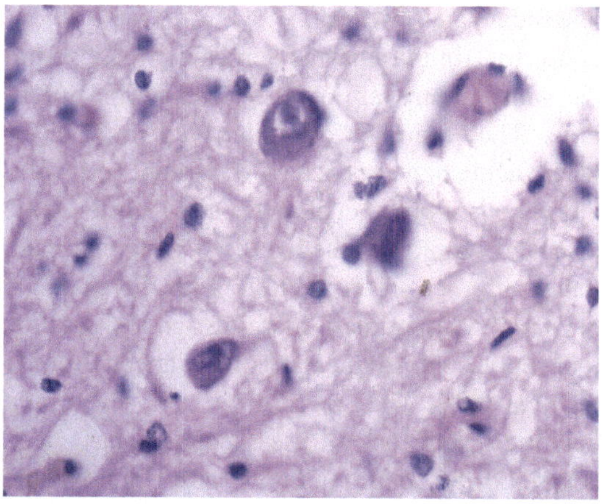

Fig. 6.15 Necrotic encephalitis with intranuclear basophilic inclusions in inborn generalized herpes infection. H-E ×600

With a longer duration of the process, necrotic meningoencephalitis occurs with widespread foci of necrosis mainly in the subependimar zones and in the frontal lobes. Cell changes identical to those described above are taking place around. Foci of gliosis are also identified, located mainly subependimar, more often in the area of the visual tubercles. They are represented by diffuse or perivascular clusters of poorly differentiated glial cells. The walls of small blood vessels in the substance of the brain are often thickened due to the proliferation of the endothelium, some of the cells of which undergo giant cell transformation. Similar vascular changes are detected in other organs. Other authors who had isolated observations described areactive necrosis, necrosis with perifocal lymphoplasmocytic infiltration, foci of gliosis, more often periventricular, swelling of the cytoplasm of neurons, degenerative changes in them with eosinophilic intracellular inclusions.

Similar changes are detected in the adrenal glands. In their cortex, foci of reactive necrosis are visible with the presence of large cells with a hyperchromic nucleus in the preserved organ tissue, the marginal location of chromatin in it and the presence of eosinophilic and basophilic inclusions. Macroscopically, they are small yellowish-gray foci, often surrounded by a hemorrhage zone.

Kidney changes are also often observed. Nephrothelial cells undergo a transformation characteristic of herpes. With the greatest severity of the process, necrotic changes in the epithelium are noted, as well as circulatory disorders.

In the mucous membrane of the digestive tract, especially the esophagus, there are changes with the metamorphosis of part of the epithelial cell's characteristic of this disease and the fine-grained decay of the nuclei of these cells. Sometimes ulcers and (or) erosions occur with perifocal edema, but without a distinct cellular inflammatory reaction.

There is no information about skin lesions in most works. Were described intraepithelial vesicles with acantholysis, peeling of the surface layers of the epidermis and the presence of characteristic intracellular inclusions in epithelial cells. There are also separate works describing eye lesions.

Giant cell myocarditis, necrotic vasculitis of the pulmonary and pancreatic arteries with the presence of characteristic inclusions under light and electron microscopy are possible in the cardiovascular system.

The state of the organs of immunogenesis has been little studied. According to our data, the mass of the thymus is usually reduced, premature fatty metamorphosis or accidental transformation of an immature type are possible. Small follicles without light centers are identified in the spleen, and necrosis foci with the presence of intracellular inclusions may appear in the spleen.

We (P. V. Antonov, V. A. Zinserling, S. P. Vydumkina) conducted special studies of chronic course of herpes encephalitis. The subjects of the study were CNS tissues (brain matter, soft meninges, choroidal plexuses), CSF, and blood serum of 22 deceased children aged 1 month to 3 years with clinically unrecognized herpetic infection. All major parts of the brain were examined: the cortex and the periventricular parts of the major hemispheres in various lobes, the basal ganglia, the hippocampus, the thalamus, the brainstem (medulla oblongata and midbrain), and the cerebellum (cortex and dentate nucleus). In 17 cases, the afterbirth of deceased children was examined.

Most of the children from the neonatal period suffered from persistent neurological pathology of varying severity.

Many children had an unfavorable medical history, including the obstetric and gynecological history of their mothers.

In all the observations, an IF study of smears from the soft meninges of the cerebral hemispheres and vascular plexuses, serological examination of blood serum and cerebrospinal fluid (complement binding reaction), as well as macroscopic and microscopic (cytological and histological) examination of CNS tissues was performed. In 20 cases, an IHC study was conducted with the detection of HSV 1/2 antigen.

The results of the virological examination according to at least one method were positive in all cases.

Microscopic examination revealed a number of changes that were considered specific for the HSV lesion. First of all, these were oxyphilic and basophilic intracranial inclusions, of which the latter were often surrounded by a rim of enlightenment. In many cells, hyperchromatosis and enlargement of the nuclei were noted, their uneven color, matte appearance, often chromatin was located in large clumps, often on the periphery of the nuclei. The described inclusions were detected in different cells of the central nervous system meningocytes, in the epithelium of the vascular plexus, ependymocytes, endotheliocytes. Often the inclusions were localized in the cerebral cortex, less often, but also quite regularly, in the basal ganglia, thalamus, and even less often in the brain stem and cerebellum. Inflammatory infiltrates were identified, consisting mainly of lymphocytes, occasionally with an admixture of histiocytes. In the meninges, they were, as a rule, focal or small-focal in nature, in some cases, they were located over a fairly large length, while sometimes there were areas of fibroblastic changes. The cell concentration was low. Also, weakly or moderately pronounced infiltration was detected in the vessel walls and perivascularly (Fig. 6.16), sometimes it was accompanied by vascular fibrosis, swelling and proliferation of endothelial cells. Most often, such changes occurred in vessels of medium and small calibers, usually arteries and arterioles, less often—veins. Their localization was diverse (including the brainstem and cerebellum), but still somewhat more common in the cerebral cortex. Separate infiltrates and focal fibrosis were also observed in the vascular plexus tissue.

In most cases, gliosis of brain tissue was detected. Often it was located in sub-perpendicular sections, representing a narrow or wider band. Sometimes focal and diffuse-focal gliosis was detected in the deep layers of the large hemispheres, the size of the foci ranged from 50 to 100 μm. Often, the glial elements were located near or close to the blood vessels (Fig. 6.16). In some cases, gliosis was mainly found in the basal

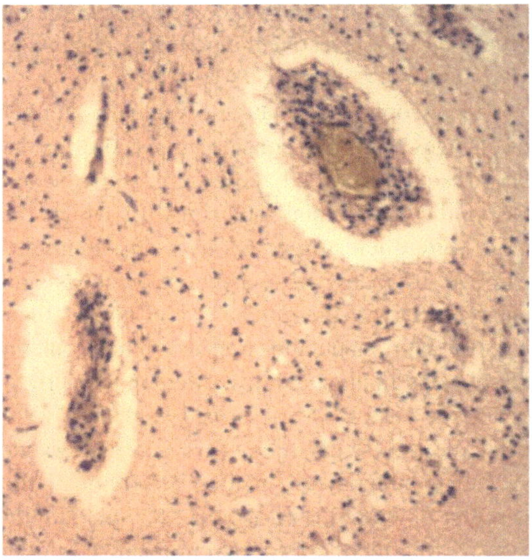

Fig. 6.16 Productive vasculitis in chronic herpes encephalitis

ganglia, thalamus, hippocampus, in others-in the cortical and subcortical parts of the brain.

In many observations, changes in the ependyma were found in the form of its folding, often quite deep and on some sections having the appearance of small cysts lined with ependymocytes. The study of serial sections convincingly showed that these are ependymal folds. In addition, small calcifications, increased satellite formation, often with separate neuronophagic nodules, and a violation of the cytoarchitectonics of the cerebral cortex were also detected. The described changes occurred in all cases, but their frequency and severity tended to be directly related to the severity of the clinical picture. There was no convincing correlation with the age of children; in different age groups, there was either an active process (intracranial inclusions, vasculitis) or a torpid current (gliosis). This circumstance may indicate that the persistence of viruses proceeds in waves. Changes typical for herpetic infection were found in all the studied afterbirths in varying degrees of severity. The presence of such changes in the afterbirth confirms the fact of intrauterine infection of the studied children. The presence of antibodies not only in the blood serum, but also in the cerebrospinal fluid strongly indicates both the duration of the infectious process and the localization of the antigens of these viruses within the central nervous system. In the IHC study, which detected replicating viruses, HSV antigens were detected mainly during active infection or its activation in the walls of blood vessels, on the surface of blood cells, soft meninges, single nerve, and glial cells. In the area of glial nodules, the virus antigen was not detected in any observation. Taken together, the described changes can be considered as manifestations of a weakly (rarely moderately) pronounced inflammatory reaction caused by HSV. There were no fundamental differences in the morphological picture in HSV types 1 and 2. Thus, it can be assumed that herpes simplex viruses of types 1 and 2, which infected the fetal central nervous system in utero, can persist for a long time, causing typical morphological changes; the course of such an infectious process is undulating. The persistence of HSV in the central nervous system is often accompanied by clinical manifestations similar to those described in encephalopathy and cerebral palsy in children, since most of the detected morphological changes indicate a viral lesion of the central nervous system and correlate with the severity of the clinical picture; changes associated with other etiological factors of neurological pathology were significantly less pronounced. However, pathogenesis of such lesions require further study.

The pathogenesis of herpes infection was also studied in experimental studies on mice with intravaginal infection, on rabbits using various methods of infection: introduction of the virus onto the scarified cornea, intravenously, and intraperitoneal.

6.4 Cytomegalovirus Infection

Cytomegalovirus (CMV) (herpes virus 5) has been known as pathogen causing different lesions, especially in newborns with immunodeficiency, patient with HIV infection in AIDS stage and transplantations for decades. Virus is able to persist and cause acute replicative infection of different cell populations in immunodeficiency state. Typical "owl eye" intranuclear inclusions pathognomic for active infection are widely known.

Cytomegalovirus is a DNA virus belonging to the Betaherpesvirinae subfamily of Herpesviridae family. Congenital CMV infection, more frequent in cases of poor socioeconomic status, may have serious clinical consequences [81–83]. Considering the relatively high number of CMV seronegative women of reproductive age, the risk of primary CMV infection during gestation is relevant [84]. Moreover, unlike other infectious diseases, the risk of fetal involvement from CMV infection in pregnancy is greater in the population, as the prevalence of serological positivity in women of childbearing age is high. Specific antibodies to CMV among pregnant women are determined in 40% of cases in developed countries and up to 100% in developing countries [85–88]. The frequency of congenital cytomegalovirus infection according to Mussi-Pinhata et al. [89] is 1.08%. CMV after a first infection can cause reactivations in the pregnant woman, being able to determine fetal infection [90]. In this last situation, the probability of CMV transmission to the fetus is lower than in the course of the first maternal infection. The transplacental transmission of human CMV infection during pregnancy is about 20–70% during the primary maternal infections, while the risk of transmission/disease is lower as 1–1.5% in case of recurrent infection [91]. Transmission may occur throughout the whole pregnancy period, but mainly in the first trimester, coming into contact with body fluids (such as saliva, urine, blood, and genital secretions) from an infected individual [92].

The study by Kvitkina [93] presents one of the variants of the pathogenesis of placental insufficiency, asphyxia of the fetus and newborn in mothers with herpes virus infection in association with cytomegalovirus, opportunistic and chlamydial infections. It consists in the development of hemic and tissue hypoxia in the body of a pregnant woman due to the inhibition of erythropoiesis and the functional activity of erythrocytes in terms of gas transport function (stage I), the flow of low-oxygenated blood into the intervillous space and a decrease in the volume of released oxygen, as the causes of the development of chronic respiratory failure of the placenta (stage II), the development of fetal hypoxia, established in terms of its gas transport function (Stage III).

In observations with cytomegalovirus infection in the villous chorion both acute changes with villous necrosis and villous sclerosis are detected. In the cells of the stroma of the villi and in the cells of Langhans, giant cell metamorphosis of the "owl's eye" type was noted (Fig. 6.17) with a positive immunohistochemical reaction with antibodies to cytomegalovirus (Fig. 6.18). In basal plate detected lymphoplasmacytic infiltration, especially near blood vessels (Fig. 6.19) [57].

In the presence of CMV in cervical and vaginal secretions, up to 5–7% of newborns are intra-

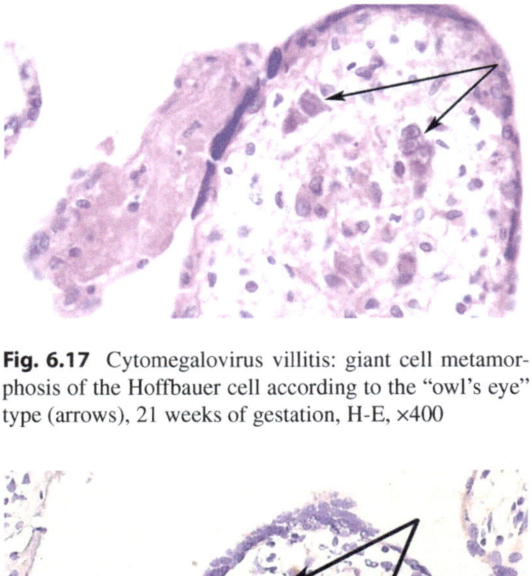

Fig. 6.17 Cytomegalovirus villitis: giant cell metamorphosis of the Hoffbauer cell according to the "owl's eye" type (arrows), 21 weeks of gestation, H-E, ×400

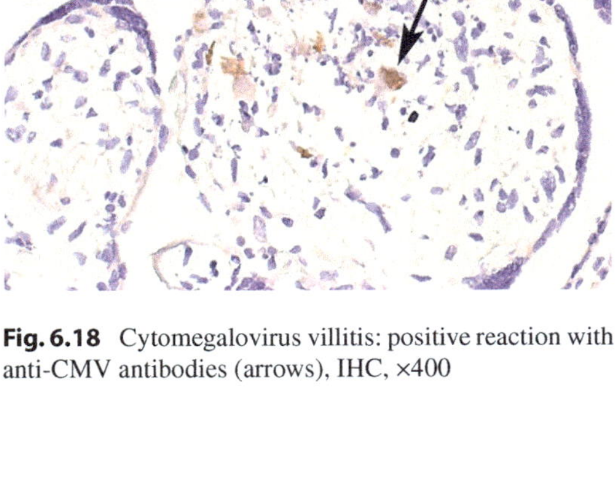

Fig. 6.18 Cytomegalovirus villitis: positive reaction with anti-CMV antibodies (arrows), IHC, ×400

natally infected. Thirty-four percent of prenatally infected children are born prematurely, with 11% of newborns having clinical signs of the disease [87]. Ten to 15% of infected neonates become symptomatic early after birth. Symptoms of CMV infection detectable already at birth include intrauterine growth retardation (IUGR), purpura, jaundice, hepatosplenomegaly, microcephaly, hearing impairment, and thrombocytopenia [94]. About 40–60% of cases symptomatic at birth subsequently develop long-term sequelae (neurological disorders, vision and hear loss) [82, 83]. In contrast, childhood sequelae developing after an asymptomatic early postnatal period occur in 10–15% of cases, and mostly include progressive hearing loss [95].

Typical cytomegalic changes ("owl's eye") can be detected both in many organs, which is designated by the term "generalized cytomegaly," and in some of them, "localized cytomegaly." The latter refers to the salivary glands (cytomegalic sialadenitis) (Fig. 6.20) [36].

The organs of the genitourinary system are also relatively often affected. The most typical localization of cytomegalic cells is the epithelium of the proximal tubules; less often, similar changes occur in the epithelium of the collecting ducts, the endothelium of the capillaries of the renal corpuscles and the epithelium of the capsules (Fig. 6.21). Occasionally, epithelial cells of the urinary tract undergo the same metamorphosis. The degree of lymphohistiocytic infiltration varies widely, but it is usually insignificant.

In inborne CMV infection can develop lesions of other organs as well, including thyroid (Fig. 6.22) and CNS. The development of productive necrotic meningoencephalitis is charac-

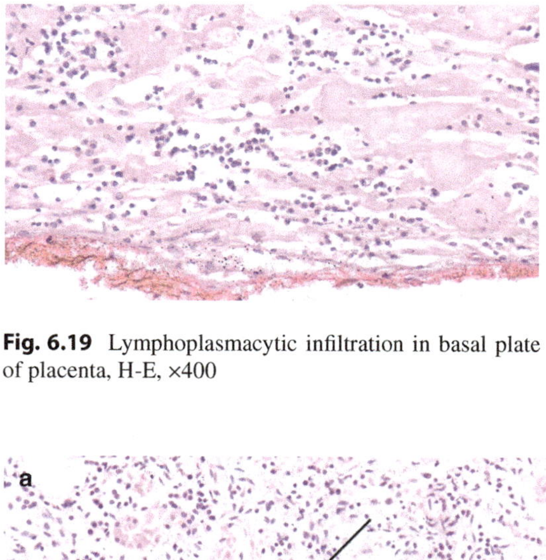

Fig. 6.19 Lymphoplasmacytic infiltration in basal plate of placenta, H-E, ×400

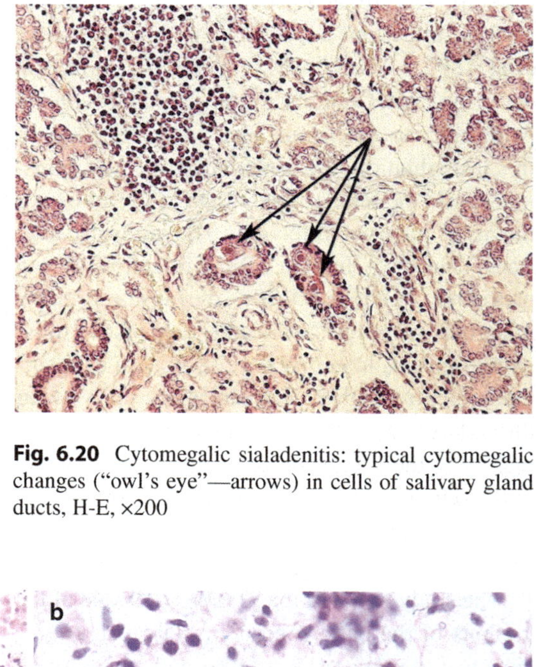

Fig. 6.20 Cytomegalic sialadenitis: typical cytomegalic changes ("owl's eye"—arrows) in cells of salivary gland ducts, H-E, ×200

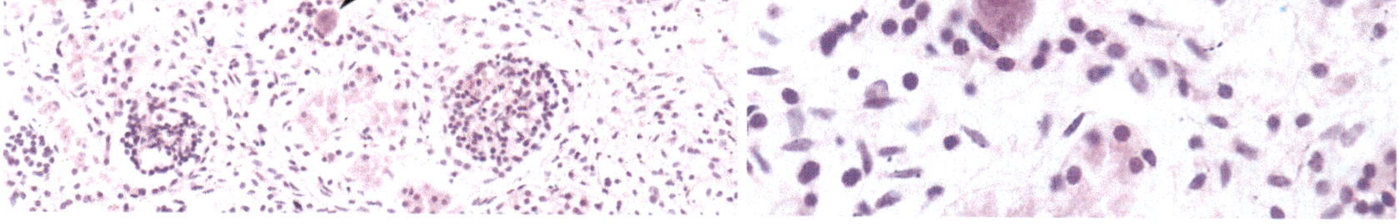

Fig. 6.21 Cytomegalovirus giant cell metamorphosis according to the "owl's eye" type (arrow), kidney of fetus of 21 weeks of gestation, H-E, (**a**) ×200; (**b**) ×1000

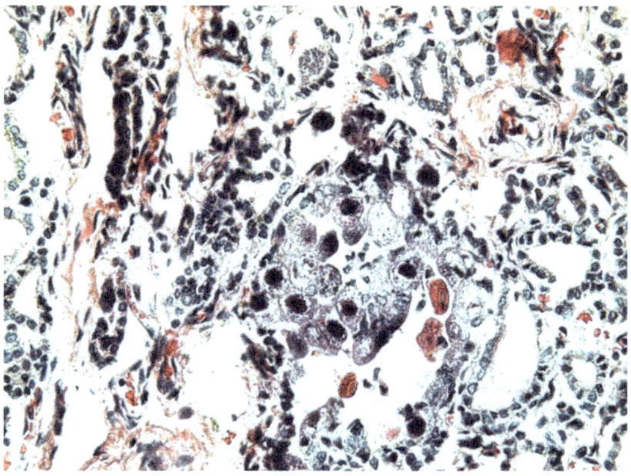

Fig. 6.22 Typical CMV lesion of thyroid. H-E ×400

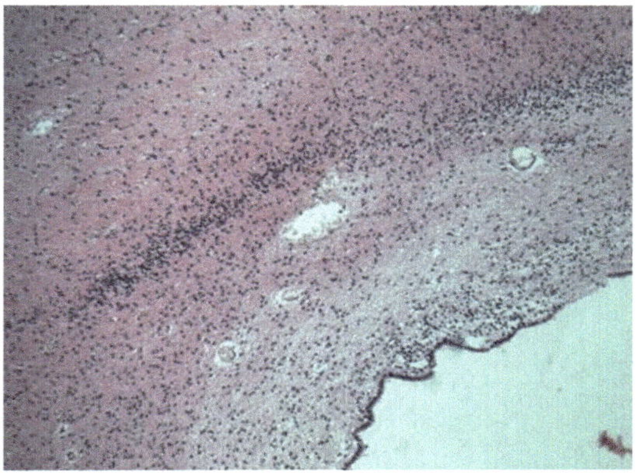

Fig. 6.23 Subependymal gliosis in intrauterine cytomegaly H-E ×100

teristic. Following variants of lesions are distinguished as well: damage to the vessel wall, ischemia, leukomalacia, deposition of calcium salts until the formation of mineralizing vasculopathy, defeat of the germinal matrix, violation of neuronal migration with the development of lissencephalopathy, polymicrogyria, ependymitis, water pipe stenosis with hydrocephalus, subependicular cysts (Fig. 6.23), and proliferation of meninges (Fig. 6.24). Often the damage is caused by indirect exposure to toxins-necrosis, cysts, calcium deposition, atrophy, leukoencephalopathy. If infection occurs in the 1–2 trimester, then the formation of malformations of development, the deposition of calcium salts is typical. During infection in the first trimester, the formation of destructive changes, calcification, and ventricular dilatation were observed.

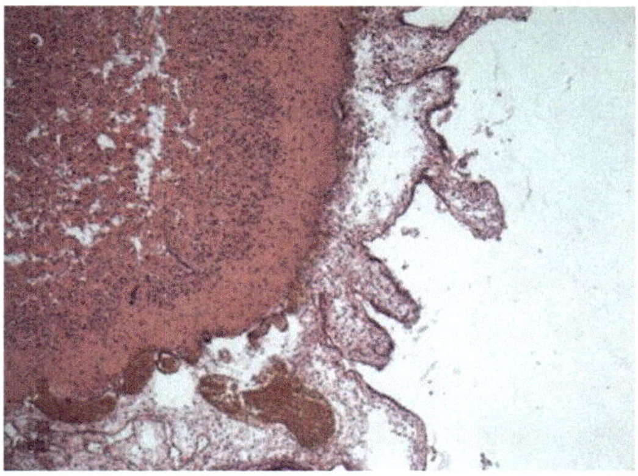

Fig. 6.24 Proliferation of soft meninges in intrauterine cytomegaly H-E ×100

6.5 Epstein-Barr Virus Infection

Epstein–Barr virus (EBV) belongs to the Herpesviridae family (type 4 herpes) and is capable of causing both acute and chronic infectious lesions, autoimmune reactions and is a generally recognized oncogenic agent.

Christian et al. [96] hypothesized that EBV antibody titers would be greater with increasing gestational age due to suppression of cell-mediated immune function. As an opportunistic latent virus, factors inducing immunosuppression allow EBV to reactivate. Reactivation can be associated with the release of viral antigens and complete infectious virus particles, resulting in the initiation of an antibody response. Thus, EBV VCA IgG antibody titers can provide an indirect measure of cell-mediated immune function [96]. The most common complications of pregnancy in cases of EBV infection are preterm birth and intrauterine growth retardation syndrome.

When the placenta is damaged by the EBV, chorionic villi against the background of impaired branching and differentiation show signs of productive non-specific villitis with lymphocytic infiltration (Fig. 6.25) and with IHC-positive cells with Epstein–Barr virus (Fig. 6.26) [97].

In study Kim et al. [98], positive staining for EBER1 was limited to glandular epithelial cells in the decidua with no other type of cells demonstrating positivity. Expression of EBNA1, LMP1, and RPMS1 was confirmed alongside EBER1 expres-

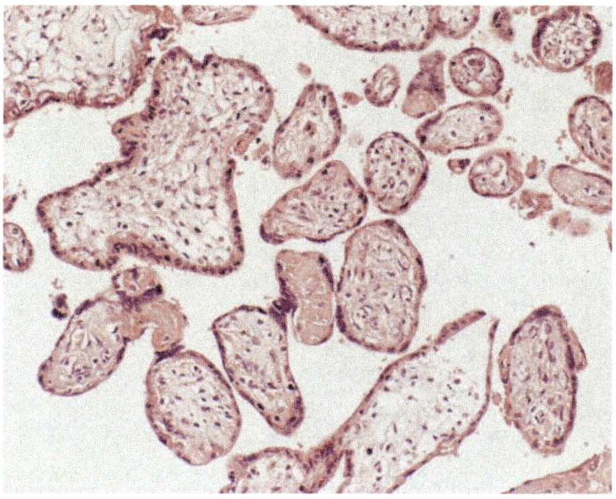

Fig. 6.25 EBV placentitis, 29 weeks of gestation; H&E, ×200

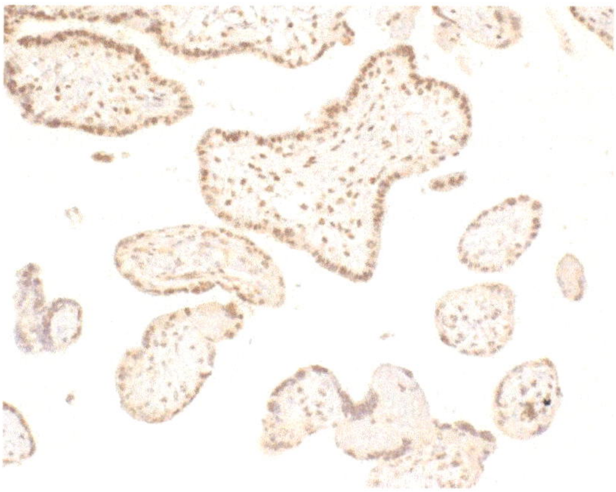

Fig. 6.26 EBV-positive cells in placenta, IHC, ×200

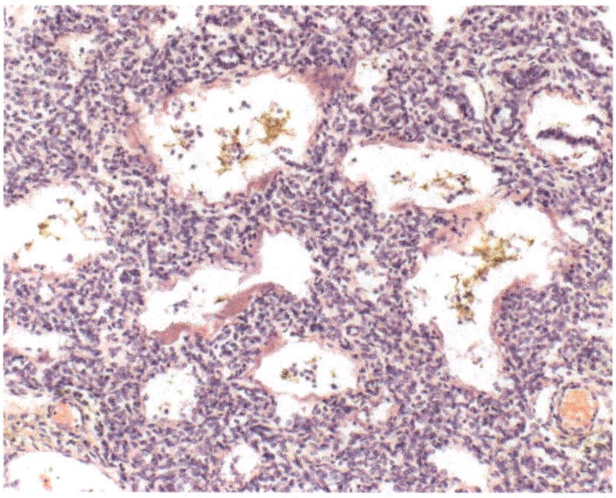

Fig. 6.27 Lung lesion in a case of intrauterine EBV infection; H-E, ×100

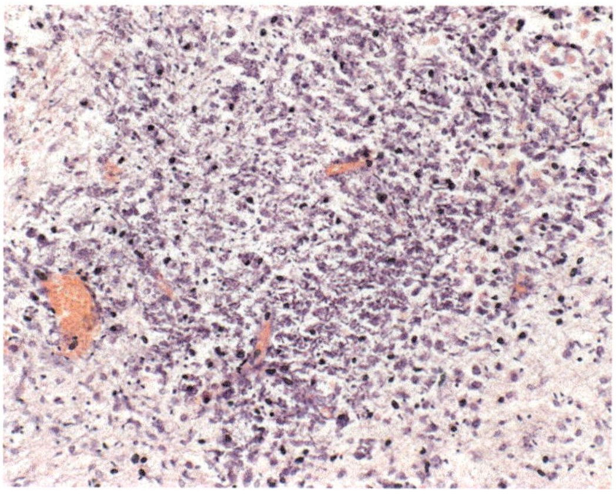

Fig. 6.28 EBV necrotic encephalitis in the same case; H-E, ×200

sion, further confirming latent EBV infection. EBV-positive cells had a distinct morphology that could be distinguished not only from EBV-negative cells of EBV-uninfected cases but also EBV-negative cells of EBV-infected placenta. The nuclei of EBV-positive cells were larger, longer, rounder, had a less condensed chromatin, and had more abundant cytoplasm compared with those of EBV-negative cells. Interestingly, acute or chronic placental inflammations were not associated with EBV gene expression. Moreover, amniotic epithelial cells that has been used to transfer EBV under experimental conditions in the past did not express EBV latent genes even in EBV-infected placentas. CD21 is a cellular receptor for the EBV entry into human B cells. However, cellular receptor for epithelial cell is not well recognized. We examined the expression of CD21 in the placenta, and confirmed that all the fetal and maternal cells in the placenta including EBV-positive cells did not express CD21 [98].

We report [97] of the case of vertical EBV infection with damage of lungs and encephalitis. This is a case of an infant girl born at 29 weeks gestational age. EBV-specific immunostains (Novocastra) were studied.

Birth weight was 1500 g, died 8 h after birth. The lungs histology demonstrates the presence of respiratory distress syndrome and viral pneumonia with lymphocytic invasion (Fig. 6.27). In brain was shown lymphohistocytic inflammation and focal necrosis (Fig. 6.28). In liver was shown lymphohistocytic inflammation and cells with hyperchromic nuclei (Fig. 6.29).

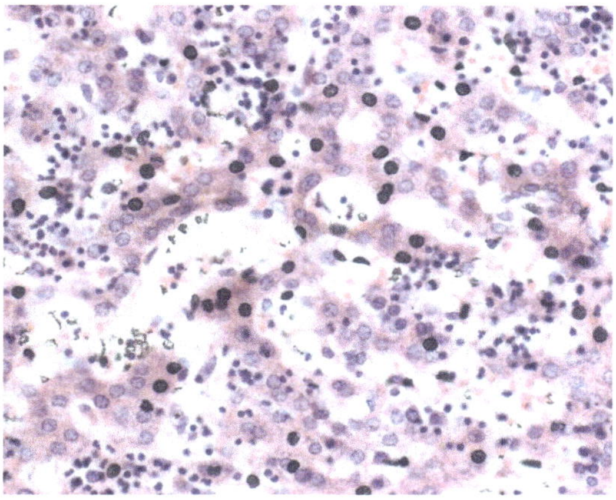

Fig. 6.29 Liver changes in the same case. Mononeclear infiltration and hyperchromic nuclei; H&E, ×200

The placenta's weight was 300 g. Macroscopic placental examination shows slight and unspecific changes.

Histology demonstrated chronic villitis with lymphocytic invasion. EBV-specific immunostains with brain, lung, liver, and placenta were studied and were positive (Fig. 6.30).

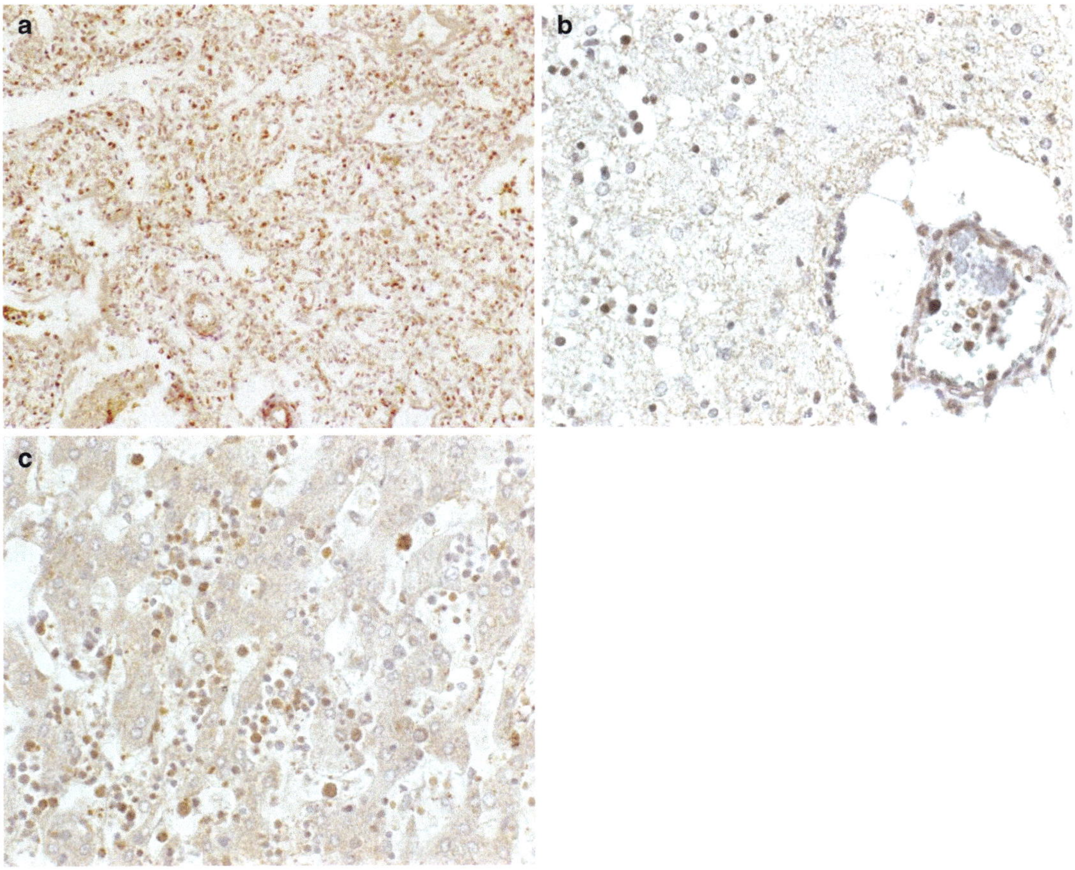

Fig. 6.30 EBV-positive cells in lung (**a**), brain (**b**) ×200, and liver (**c**) ×400; IHC

6.6 Parvovirus B19 Infection

Parvovirus B19, a DNA-containing virus, was classified as an erythrovirus in 1995 and renamed "B19 virus" or "B19V.". It has been established that the frequency of infection of pregnant women with B19V is approximately 1 case per 400 pregnancies. The most typical clinical manifestation of parvovirus B19 infection is erythema infectiosum (also known as "slap syndrome" or "fifth disease") [99]. At the same time, it has been shown that in most pregnant women the infection is asymptomatic, but it can lead to damage to the organs of the fetus—this usually occurs between 20 and 28 weeks of intrauterine development. Parvovirus B19 vertical transmission occurs in about 30% of cases of maternal infection [100]. For instance, acute congenital B19V infection in pregnancy results in non-immune hydrops fetalis and fetal death [101]. Fetuses at first and second trimester are most susceptible because erythroid precursor development is predominant at these stages [102]. Ultimately, parvovirus infection can lead to intrauterine fetal death in the second trimester or stillbirth. Fetal death usually occurs 4–6 weeks after maternal infection with parvovirus B19 [3].

Differentiating syncytiothrophoblast and cytotrophoblast cells have a key role in B19V vertical transmission, because of a strong expression of globoside-receptor on their surfaces. Although they are not permissive to viral infection, a receptor-mediated transcytosis process leads to release of the virus into fetal circulation [103]. Fetal capillary endothelium in placental villi could also be an additional target of B19V, leading to a structural and functional injury concurring to anomalous maternal-fetal blood exchanges and to the dissemination of the virus [100]. Furthermore, B19V infection of EPCs generates a DNA damage response by interfering with repair pathways and thus promoting viral DNA replication [104].

Macroscopically, the placenta is usually hyperplastic. Histological examination against the background of hydropic changes shows a pronounced immaturity of the villi with perivillous fibrinoid deposits (Fig. 6.31). The villus stroma is infiltrated with mononuclear leukocytes. In the lumen of the vessels of the villi and in the stromal canals, specific cells called "Chinese lantern" are detected. An immunohistochemical study showed a positive reaction in cells infected with B19V (Fig. 6.32) [105].

Once in the fetal circulation, the virus may then spread to fetal erythroid precursor cells (EPCs) in the liver and/or in bone marrow, and eventually cardiomyocytes, in the absence of an effective fetal immune response. The fetus is also more vulnerable considering that the half-life of its red blood cells is short (50–75 days) [106].

Here is our own observation of intrauterine parvovirus infection.

Patient V, 18 years old. At 12 weeks of pregnancy, she was hospitalized with a diagnosis of "threatened miscarriage," and conservative therapy was carried out. Ultrasound data from 02/20/12—pregnancy 19/20 weeks; fetus corresponds to the gestational age. Placenta was 21 mm thick is located on the back wall, has I degree of maturity.

On March 11, 2012, she was delivered to the maternity hospital by an ambulance with a diagnosis of:

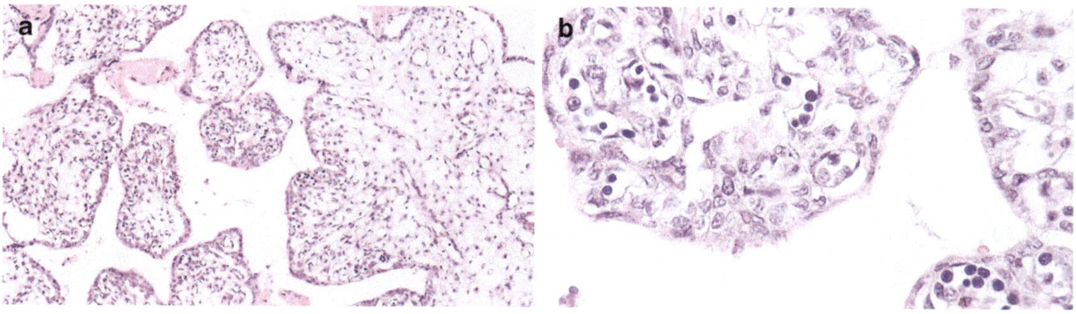

Fig. 6.31 Parvovirus B19 placentitis, 21 weeks of gestation: (**a**) ×10, (**b**) ×400; H&E

21/22 weeks' pregnancy. Threatened late miscarriage. Gestational pyelonephritis. Chronic nicotine intoxication. Burdened obstetric and gynecological history.

An ultrasound examination dated March 12, 2012 revealed congenital malformations of the fetus (hydrothorax, hydropericardium, fetal dropsy). On 03/20/2012, the fetal heartbeat was not heard, and therefore an artificial termination of pregnancy was performed for medical reasons.

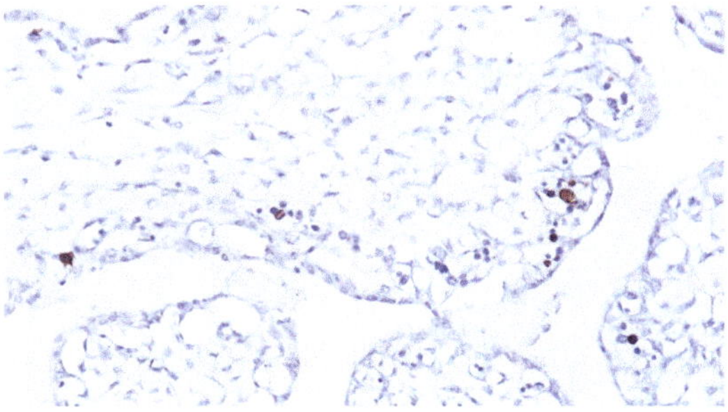

Fig. 6.32 PARVO positive cells in placenta, IHC, ×400

An autopsy study of a fetus with a body weight of 630 g and a body length of 28 cm showed signs of subcutaneous adipose tissue edema and ascites (abdominal circumference—24 cm). An internal examination in the pleural and abdominal cavities revealed a free transparent liquid of a light yellow color. The lungs are hypoplastic, with a total weight of 7 g. The liver has an uneven surface. The rest of the organs are without visible changes.

Histological examination, against the background of edematous changes, revealed cells specific for B19V infections "Chinese lantern"—compared with festive lanterns among Buddhists) in the kidneys, lungs, and myocardium. In addition, focal infiltration of mononuclear cellular elements—lymphocytes, macrophages—was noted in the myocardium.

Immunohistochemical (IHC) examination of the tissues of the above organs with polyclonal NCL-PARVO antibodies (Novocastra) showed a positive reaction in cells infected with B19V (Figs. 6.33, 6.34, and 6.35) [107].

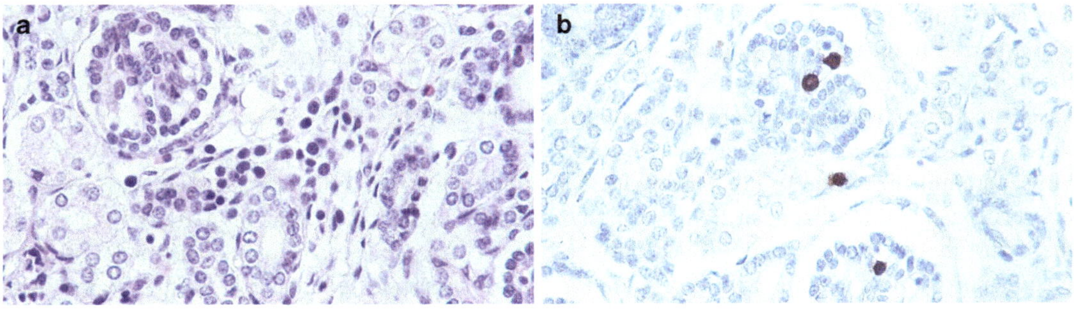

Fig. 6.33 (**a**) Parvovirus B19 in cells of kidney, H-E, ×400 (**b**) PARVO positive cells of kidney, IHC, ×400

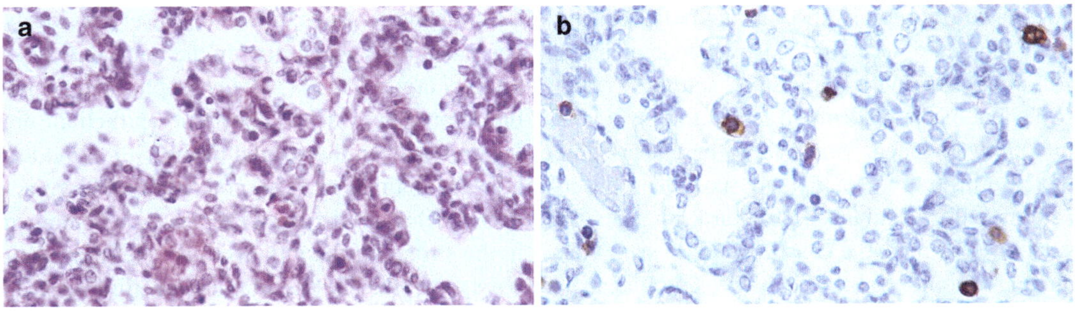

Fig. 6.34 (**a**) Parvovirus B19 in cells of lung, H-E, ×400. (**b**) PARVO positive cells of lung, IHC, ×400

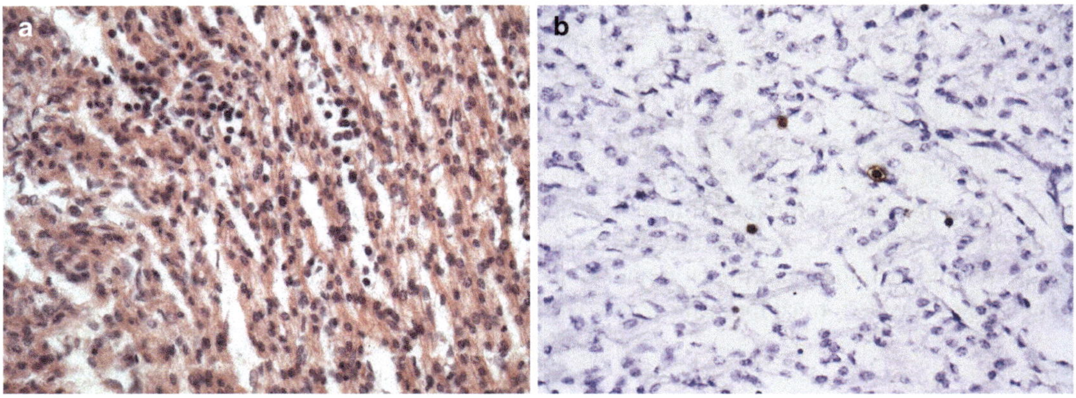

Fig. 6.35 (**a**) Parvovirus B19 myocarditis, H-E, ×200. (**b**) PARVO positive cells of myocardium, IHC, ×200

6.7 Respiratory Syncytial Virus Infection

Respiratory syncytial virus (RSV) is a leading cause of under-5 morbidity and mortality, causing an estimated 48,000–74,500 under-5 childhood deaths in 2015, 50% occurring during the first 6 months of life [108]. An inverse association has been reported between maternal RSV neutralizing antibodies and risk for RSV hospitalization among young infants [109–111]. A major barrier to the effective diagnosis of RSV is the inability to make the diagnosis solely on the basis of clinical features, which are similar to those of infections caused by adenovirus, rhinovirus, parainfluenza virus, or influenza virus. The reference standard for diagnosis (i.e., isolation of the virus in cell culture and identification of plaque morphologic features with syncytium formation) is time consuming and expensive. More recently, PCR-based testing has become more available and allows for a more rapid and specific diagnosis. Laboratory testing has only recently been adopted in academic hospital centers and is still underused in the community setting [112].

Defeat of the placenta in respiratory syncytial infection. In recent years, there has been some increase in its frequency, there have been observations with pronounced structural changes. In such observations, the cells increase in size, their nuclei become light, the wide cytoplasm is slightly acidophilic. A significant part of the cells have two or more nuclei, sometimes they form

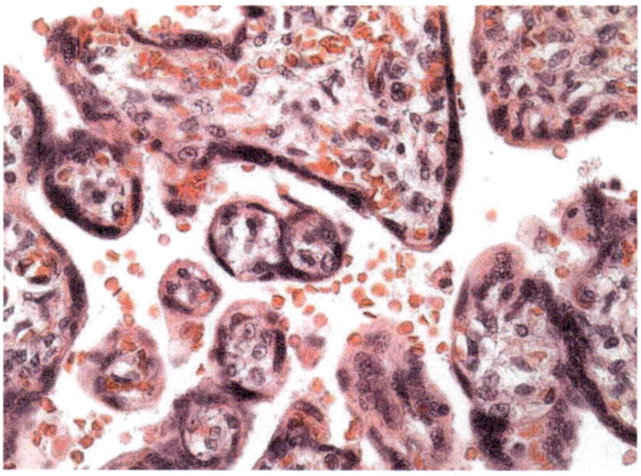

Fig. 6.36 Placenta lesion by RS-virus. Note growths of trophoblast. H-E ×600

multinucleated symplasts, similar with those in lungs. In the trophoblast, large focal growths that look like papillae are found. The nuclei of these formations are light, the cytoplasm is slightly acidophilic, extensive. The same transformation occurs in the trophoblastic islands of the intervillous space (Fig. 6.36). It should be noted that such changes are similar to those previously described by A. Zinserling in the lungs and other internal organs [113, 114]. Dystrophic and necrobiotic processes in the chorionic epithelium are insignificant. In the stroma of the villi, a moderate or sometimes more significant fibroblast reaction is detected, the nuclei of the cells contained in the stroma of the villi also become light, their sizes increase. The vascular endothelium appears swollen, the nuclei of endotheliocytes become light, sometimes endothelial cells are arranged in several rows. Inflammatory infiltration is focal in nature, partly located around the vessels and consists mainly of lymphocytes [115].

6.8 Coronavirus Disease 2019 (COVID-19)

COVID-19 caused by the severe acute respiratory syndrome coronavirus 2 (SARS-CoV-2) virus has been implicated in the clinical pathology of multiple organs and organ systems. COVID-19 has been associated with a large debate concerning the occurrence of transplacental transmission [116]. Although no transplacental transmission was reported from China, Hosier et al., presented for the first time the case of woman with COVID-19 with a SARS-CoV-2 invasion of the placenta and local tissue inflammation and fibrin deposition [117]. They reported an inflammatory infiltrate of immune cells composed of CD3+ lymphocytes and CD68+ macrophages with only infection of syncytiotrophoblast cells by SARS-CoV-2 virus. The infiltration of CD68+ placenta macrophages in SARS-CoV-2 infected placenta was next confirmed [118, 119] associated with a M2 phenotype in a case report of an asymptomatic COVID-19 positive woman [120]. Interestingly, Facchetti et al. reported a strong expression of S-protein in areas with dense monocytes-macrophage inflammation, which suggests a local activation of these cells. Thus, to date, although the presence of placental macrophage into placenta lesions was clearly established, their role in SARS-CoV-2 infection of the placenta remains to elucidate.

The localization of SARS-CoV-2 receptors, proteases, and genes involved in coding proteins that drive viral pathogenesis in the placenta predisposes the placenta to SARS-CoV-2 infection variably in all pregnancy trimesters, with antecedent placental pathology. There is a need for further studies to explicate the mechanism of entry and pathogenesis of SARS-CoV-2 in the placenta [121].

Placental infections may promote localized immune response, including inflammation resulting from an infection or immune-mediated response. Though not widely reported, maternal and fetal inflammatory features in COVID-19, positive placentas included acute chorioamnionitis, subchorionitis, funisitis, and umbilical cord vasculitis. In our practice, chronic infection-associated inflammatory lesions in SARS-CoV-2 infected placentas included chronic villitis with increased inflammatory lymphocytic infiltrate in the absence of other morbidities and chronic intervillositis with T-lymphocytes and macrophages infiltrate associated with viral RNA. Immune or idiopathic inflammatory features (villitis of unknown etiology (VUE) and associated lesions such as chronic chorioamnionitis, chronic villitis, and lymphoplasmacytic deciduitis were reported in placentas positive for SARS-CoV-2. In our practice, we describe chronic intervillositis with lymphocytes and macrophages infiltrate, perivillouse fibrinoid deposition, and villous infarction (Figs. 6.37, 6.38, and 6.39).

We made special investigation in SP Botkin infectious hospital. The medical cards of inpatient patients were analyzed (in collaboration with Dr. M.A. Vashukova) and microscopic preparations of placentas and autopsy material of the relevant observations were revised. Macro- and microscopic examination of the afterbirth was carried out in accordance with the developments of the St. Petersburg School of Perinatology. Polyclonal rabbit antibodies to the SARS-CoV-2 nucleocapsid protein (GTX135361, GeneTex, USA) and polyclonal rabbit antibodies to the S1 subunit of spike protein (spike protein) SARS-CoV-2 (GTX135360, GeneTex, USA) were used in working dilutions of 1:500. The visualization of the reaction product was carried out using the UltraVision Quanto Detection System HRP polymer system (Thermo Scientific, USA). The optimal conditions for the immunohistochemical reaction were selected after the staining procedure of parallel sections with negative and positive controls. Histological preparations were studied using a Nikon ECLIPSE Ni-U microscope (Japan) with an ×10 eyepiece, with ×20 ×40 lenses. Our results of our own research.

The pregnant women were between the ages of 20 and 35.

Brief anamnestic data are given in Table 6.1.

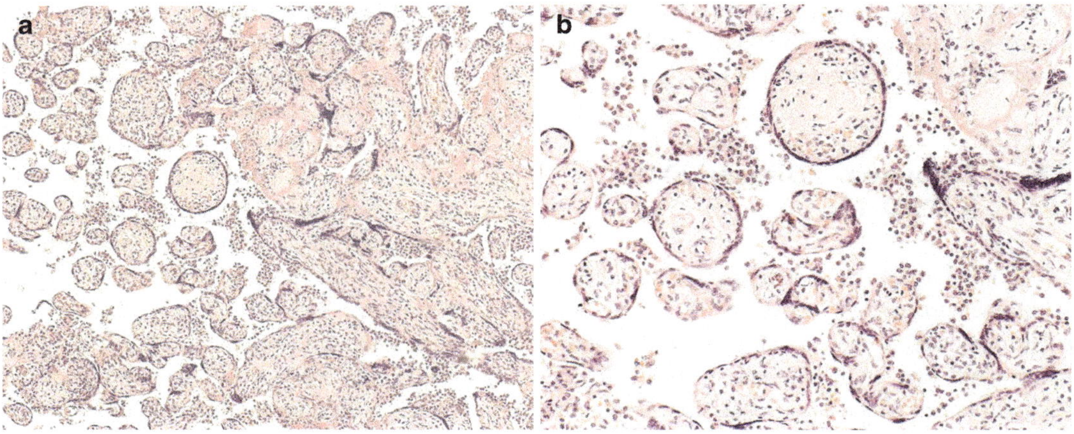

Fig. 6.37 Chronic intervillositis with lymphocytes and macrophages infiltrate in placenta with COVID-19; 20 weeks of gestation; H&E, (**a**) ×100, (**b**) ×200

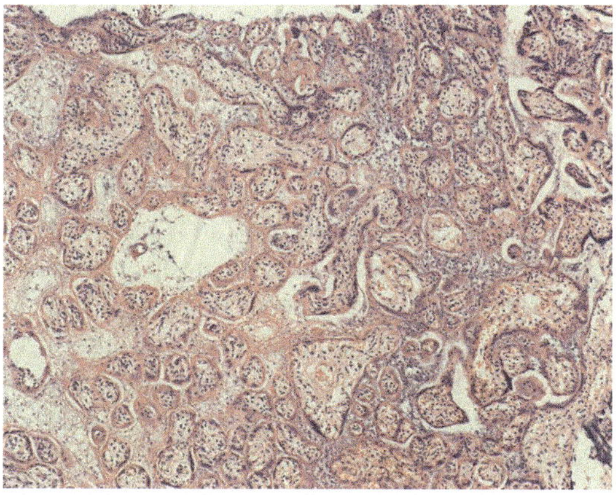

Fig. 6.38 Fibrinoid deposition around villi in placenta with COVID-19; 20 weeks of gestation; H&E, ×100

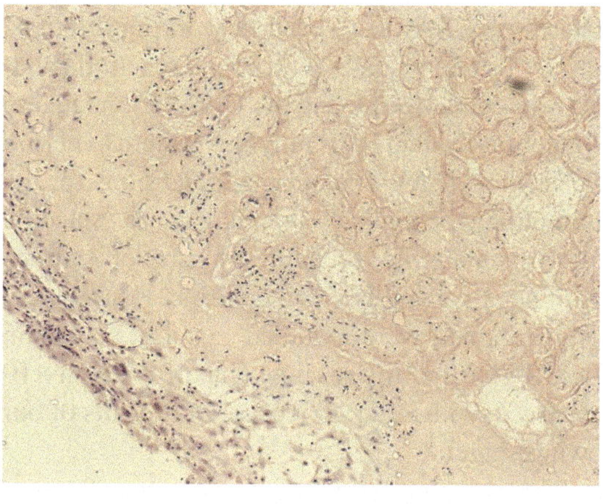

Fig. 6.39 Villous infarction, H&E, ×100

The condition of the mothers varied significantly. All women received standard therapy, in observations 1,2,6 received intensive care in the ICU, including ventilation in obs. 2.

In most cases, childbirth proceeded without complications and the condition of the newborns was highly rated on the Apgar scale (Table 6.2). The only exception was a premature baby from nab.1, who was diagnosed with SDR and transferred to a children's hospital, where his condition was stabilized after a ventilator. In two observations, the presence of early hypoglycemia was noted. In a PCR study, a positive result was obtained in only one observation (2).

Of particular interest were the outcomes studied in all observations. In two cases of premature birth, signs of immaturity of the placenta were revealed, approximately corresponding to the gestation period. In addition, all observations revealed signs of RNA viral infection, which consisted in the appearance of cells with large light nuclei, slightly altered shapes in both the maternal and fetal parts of the placenta and extraplacental membranes (Fig. 6.40a–d). In addition, it was possible to talk about the development of subcompensated chronic placental insufficiency. Syncytial buds in chorionic villi were slightly pronounced. Swelling of the nuclei of endothelial cells was noted as characteristic changes in all observations.

Table 6.1 General data related to pregnant women

No.	Initial, age	Number of pregnancy	Outcomes of previous pregnancies	Concomitant pathology	Staying in intensive care unit
1	M, 35	3	2017-cesarian section, 2010—term delivery	Not known	ICU, Art Ventil
2	Ch., 38	5	2010 delivery, 2012, 206 med abortion, 2018—planed cesarian section	Not known	ICU
3	B., 28	3	2017—in vitro fertilization death during preterm delivery, 2019—delivery	Chron. salpingooophoritis	No
4	A., 20	2	2017—preterm delivery	Not known	No
5	C., 30	5	2013, 2015—term delivery, 2016—spontaneous abortion, 2017—medical abortion	Not known	No
6	P., 35	3	2008—spontaneous abortion, 2010—delivery	Bronchial asthma, Chron. Vir. Hep C	No

Table 6.2 General data about newborns

No.	Term of delivery	Apgar scale	PCR SARS-CoV2	Diagnosis
1	31 week	1/2/2	Neg	Syndrom of respiratory distress of newborns, heavy asphyxia at delivery, inborn anemia, hypocoagulation
2	Full-term	8/9	Pos	Carrier SARS-CoV2
3	Full-term	7/9	Neg	Early neonatal hypoglycemia, trombocytosis
4	Full-term	7/8	Neg	Neonatal icterus, crevis of the hard and soft palate
5	Full-term	7/8	No data	Intrauterine hypoxia at the time of delivery
6	33 week	7/8	Neg	Early neonatal hypoglicemia

In the IHC study, both the studied antigens of the SARS-CoV-2 nucleocapsid and the S1 subunit of the spike protein (spike protein) SARS-CoV-2 were detected in moderate amounts, including in the fetal part of the afterbirth (Fig. 6.41a, b).

6.8.1 Discussion

Given the data on the ability of the new coronavirus to cause direct damage to many cells, the probability of direct damage to the afterbirth is very high. Having the long-term experience in the diagnosis of RNA viral placentitis as well as the similarity of the changes detected in the maternal and fetal parts of the afterbirth with those observed in COVID-19 in the lungs, it is highly likely to assume the ability of the new coronavirus to transplacental transport. This phenomenon is also confirmed by the results of the IHC study, in which both "nuclear" and "spike" antigens, although in small quantities, were detected in the fetal parts of the afterbirth. Negative PCR results from nasopharyngeal flushes of a newborn child do not allow us to deny the possibility of intrauterine transplacental infection, since the virus cannot immediately enter the mucous membrane of the upper respiratory tract. Nevertheless, in one of our observations, a positive PCR result was obtained.

The most important issue is the clinical relevance of the identified changes in the afterbirth. It is very likely that among the mechanisms of premature birth, coronavirus also played a significant role in our two observations. The severe condition of the child in case 1 can also be presumably associated with it. At the same time, term delivery in four cases and the absence of severe pathology in five children immediately

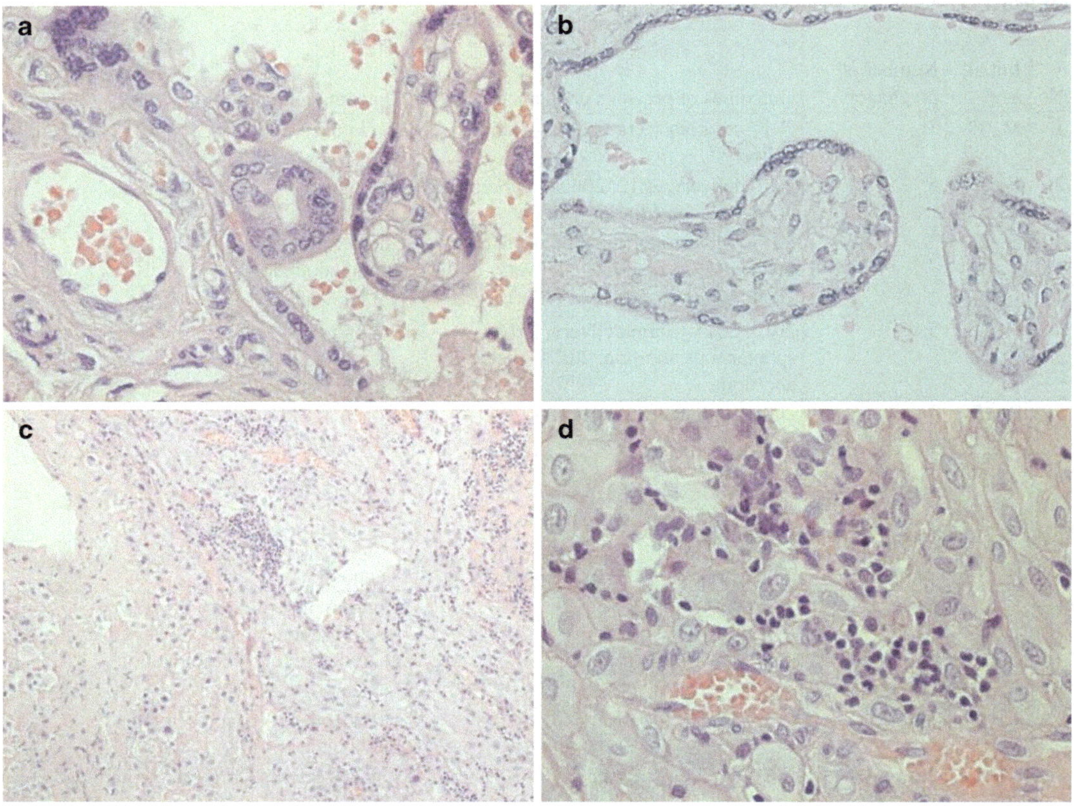

Fig. 6.40 Changes in placentas in COVID-19 infected mothers. H-E. (**a**) Immature terminal villi of the placenta in case 1. A sharp increase in the size of light syncytiotrophoblast nuclei and Hofbauer cells, characteristic of RNA viral infections, is visible. ×400. (**b**) Mature terminal villi in case. 2. A significant increase in the light nuclei of syncytiotrophoblast, characteristic of RNA viral infections, is visible. ×400. (**c**) The extraplacental membrane in the case 1. Focal mononuclear infiltration and transformation of decidual membrane cells characteristic of RNA viral infections are visible. ×100. (**d**) Similar changes. Mixed infiltration and changes in the nuclei of endothelial cells are visible. ×400

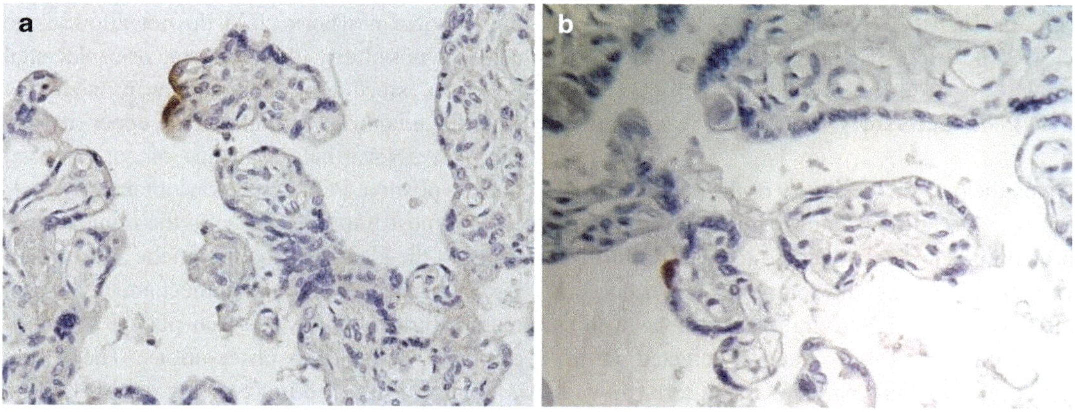

Fig. 6.41 Antigens of the SARS-Cov-2 virus in placentas during immunohistochemical examination. (**a**) "Spike" antigen in the syncytiotrophoblast of the terminal villi in nab. 6. ×100. (**b**) "Nuclear" antigen in the syncytiotrophoblast of the terminal villi in the same observation. ×100

after birth do not allow us to exclude the development of some pathological processes in these children in the future. It should not be forgotten that many representatives of the coronavirus family are capable of causing chronic infectious processes, at least in some animals. In addition, in many intrauterine infections, including those caused by RNA-containing viruses, the possibility of a low-symptom course leading to moderate impairment of psychomotor development, the development of autoimmune and other secondary diseases has been proven. The problem of perinatal COVID-19 certainly needs further study, and children are subject to observation.

6.9 Influenza Virus Infection

Influenza viruses could cause acute respiratory symptoms including fever, malaise, and coughing. Although influenza viruses are classified into A, B, C, and D types, only type A viruses, such as swine influenza (H1N1), are recognized to have a wide range of hosts including mankind and become a major driver of human infectious diseases [122]. During the 2009 pandemic of influenza A virus (IAV), pregnant women were more frequently hospitalized than individuals in the general population [123]. In addition, the maternal mortality rate of IAV infection was significantly higher in the USA, which is in line with 27–45% maternal mortality. It should be noted that the possibility of adverse maternal outcomes increases with the advancing gestational age [124]. Women with full-term pregnancy are five times more likely to be hospitalized with IAV infection than the ones at postpartum or early pregnancy stage [125].

IAV infection during pregnancy causes severe fetal and neonatal complications as well, including intrauterine growth retardation, preterm birth, neonatal death, and neurological disorders. The reasons for fetal mortality and morbidity upon IAV infection during pregnancy are currently unclear. Different from TORCH pathogens, vertical transmission of IAV appears to be rare because of infrequent viremia, despite a recent study reported that the highly pathogenic strain H5N1 could be detected in the placental trophoblasts and fetal respiratory tract [126, 127] Maternal symptoms of IAV infection, such as fever, hypoxia, and septic shock, could exert influence on fetal health in the absence of direct fetal infection. Recently, Liong et al. demonstrated virus dissemination to major maternal blood vessels leads to a peripheral "vascular storm," featured as profoundly elevated proinflammatory and antiviral mediators in the maternal vascular system, which could subsequently induce hypoxia in the placenta and fetal brain [128]. Moreover, accumulating evidence suggests that offspring born to prenatally IAV-infected mothers exposed high risk of chronic diseases in later life, among which neurocognitive disorders, autism for instance, are the best described ones [129–131]. Moreover, Jacobsen et al. proposed that neonates from IAV-infected pregnant dame exhibited increased susceptibility to viral and bacterial infections due to reduced hematopoietic development and immune responses, which further highlights the importance of fundamental mechanistic study regarding IAV induced poor maternal-fetal outcomes in the future.

According to a study by Melnikova, changes in decidual cells and trophoblast characteristic of influenza viruses are observed in the basal plates of placentas [36]. Such cells are large in size, have slightly acidophilic cytoplasm, sometimes with basophilic granularity, and large light nuclei. An immunofluorescent study revealed influenza virus antigens and fucsinophilic or cytoplasmic inclusions surrounded by a basophilic rim. Epithelial cells subsequently undergo dystrophic changes, become rounded and slough into the lumen. Damage to the basal lamina by influenza viruses of all identified strains was characterized by the development of extensive areas of acidophilic coagulation necrosis in it. Fibrin deposits are not detected in these areas. Moderate lymphocytic inflammatory infiltration is noted. In the vessels of the basal plate, perivascular infiltrates and significant destructive changes are observed in the form of endothelial swelling and disorganization of stromal fibers. This kind of change can be considered as basal deciduitis. In all placentas,

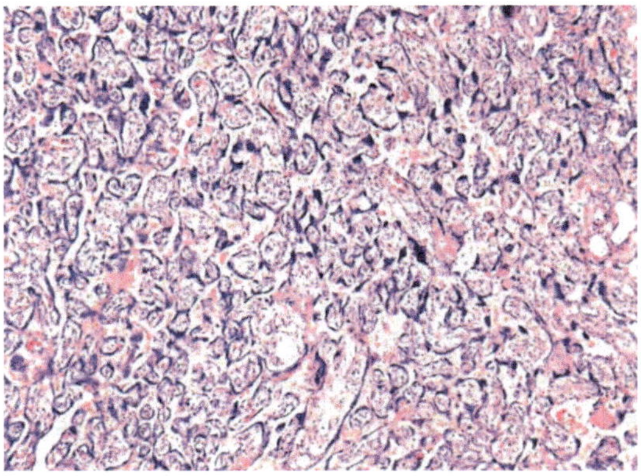

Fig. 6.42 Placenta in influenza. Disseminated lesions of villous chorion ×200

focal disseminated lesions of the villous chorion were noted (Fig. 6.42). The changes were localized in small terminal and, to a lesser extent, large and medium villi [36].

In the chorionic epithelium of the villi and trophoblast islands, they consisted of the appearance of areas with large light nuclei and extensive weakly oxyphilic cytoplasm. A specific fluorescence with influenza A and B viruses was found in them. In some places, entire villi undergo similar changes; in them, the trophoblast appears thickened, the cytoplasm becomes light, and the nuclei are arranged in several rows.

Subsequently, necrobiotic processes develop in the syncytiotrophoblast, as a result of which the cytoplasm becomes sharply acidophilic, the nuclei undergo pyknosis, and areas devoid of epithelial lining, the so-called bare villi appear.

In parallel with this, a significantly pronounced proliferation of cytotrophoblast is sometimes found in the villi, Langhans cells increase in size, their nuclei are large, light, and a significant increase in the nuclear-cytoplasmic index is noted. A pronounced fibroblastic reaction occurs in the terminal, anchor, and intermediate villi.

6.10 Zika Virus Infection

ZIKV is a single-stranded RNA virus of the Flaviviridae family, which was originally isolated from a rhesus monkey residing in Uganda. It spread globally from 2015 to 2016 and led to a Public Health Emergency of International Concern declared by the World Health Organization due to emerging neuropathogenicity such as the Guillain-Barré syndrome in adults and microcephaly in neonates, respectively [132]. Although ZIKV is initially recognized as a mosquito-borne virus predominately transmitted by Aedes, there has been a great accumulation of new evidence that ZIKV can be transmitted in many new routes, especially through sexual contact, blood transfusion, and most important of all, vertical transmission [133]. The clinical manifestations of systemic ZIKV infections during pregnancy present similar symptoms like those described in nonpregnant individuals, usually mild and self-limiting diseases, suggesting no specific maternal clinical features and increased pathogenicity in general. Nevertheless, clinical and basic investigations have shown that congenital ZIKV infection could dramatically provoke pregnancy diseases, such as miscarriage, IUGR, premature delivery, and fetal death [134, 135].

Another explanation for different vulnerabilities to ZIKV infection at different pregnancy stages is due to the gradually gained placental defense mechanisms along with the progress of pregnancy, which will be discussed in detail below. In addition, the transplacental transmission routines of ZIKV are still debatable [133]. Several cellular mechanisms may mediate the vertical transmission of ZIKV, including cell-to-cell spread within trophoblasts, para-placental routes (traversing the amino-chorion), autophagy-mediated placental transmission, ZIKV dissemination seeded from infected HBCs, and Ab dependent enhancement of ZIKV infection [136, 137]. Each of those mechanisms is unique somehow, indicating the complexity and heterogeneity of vertical transmitted ZIKV infection, which need to be further explored in future in-depth mechanistic studies. It is worthy of note that although some molecules are proposed as potential receptors or host factors for ZIKV infections in different organs, such as Axl, Tyro3, and Mertk, none of them has been validated in the setting of transplacental infection, which impedes the mechanisms underpinning strong placental tropism of ZIKV [138, 139].

In fact, malfunction of placenta alone could induce CZS-like diseases (See also: Chap. 8). Thus, whether CZS is caused by direct ZIKV infection or placental insufficiency indirectly (or combined effects) is another aspect worth pondering. Therefore, a transient ZIKV infection during pregnancy is likely to affect future development and health of the neonates and even adulthood health in a long run, which still needs in-depth mechanistic studies to address [133].

Pregnant women infected by ZIKA virus present a chronic placentitis with a chronic villous inflammation, edema and trophoblastic lesions [116, 136]. There is evidence that ZIKA infection compromises mesenchymal and Hofbauer cells in human villi [140, 141]. Immunohistochemistry approaches also reveal that ZIKA virus stimulates the proliferation of placental macrophages within the chorionic villous stroma [142]. CD163 or CD68 positive cells are colocalized with ZIKA virus antigens in vivo [137, 143]. Ex vivo models show a higher permittivity of placental macrophages to ZIKA virus than trophoblasts [144]. Recently, it has been shown that Abs directed against dengue virus increase ZIKA virus infection of Hofbauer cells, suggesting that preexisting immunity to dengue affects host response to ZIKA virus [145]. The replication of ZIKA virus within Hofbauer cells induces the production of type I IFN, IL-6, CCL3, and inducible protein (IP)-10 [146]. The blockade of IFN production using Janus Kinase (JAK) inhibitors inhibits the production and the replication of the ZIKA virus in human Hofbauer cells in vitro [147]. Additionally, the expression of the co-stimulatory molecules CD80 and CD86 by Hofbauer cells is increased, suggesting that they are potentially APCs in vivo. All these studies suggest that the primary tropism of the ZIKA virus for placental macrophages enables the virus to cross the placental barrier and to eventually access to the fetal compartment [116].

6.11 Other Viruses

In the present manual, we discussed only most common (or frequently diagnosed) perinatal virus infections. There are data that perinatal infection could develop in measles (in case of acute infection in pregnant women). Old literature presents rare cases of intrauterine German measles causing at early stage of pregnancy Gregg syndrome (see Chap. 8) and at late stages productive encephalitis, placenta is characterized by formation of multinuclear cells (Fig. 6.43). In our studies of previous decades were described single cases of placenta lesions due to parainfluenza and adenovirus. One can suppose that certain changes can occur due to other viral pathogens as well (rhinoviruses, metapneumovirus, etc.).

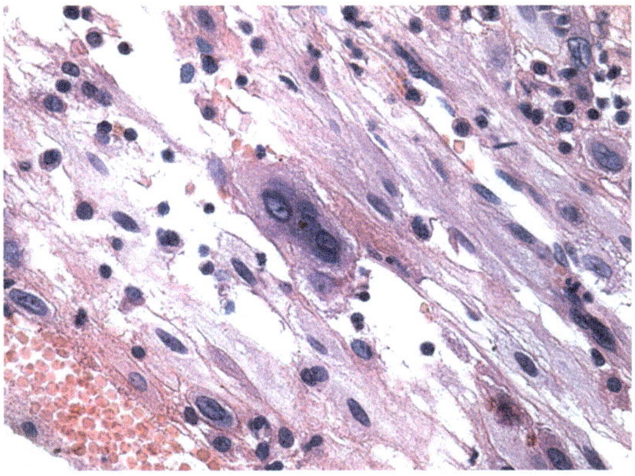

Fig. 6.43 Placenta in morbilli. Formation of multinuclear cells. H-E ×400

References

1. Magnius L, Mason WS, Taylor J, Kann M, Glebe D, Dény P, et al. ICTV virus taxonomy profile: Hepadnaviridae. J Gen Virol. 2020;101:571–2. https://doi.org/10.1099/jgv.0.001415.
2. Nwaohiri A, Schillie S, Bulterys M, Kourtis AP. Hepatitis C virus infection in children: how do prevent it and how do we treat it? Expert Rev Anti Infect Ther. 2018;16:689–94. https://doi.org/10.1080/14787210.2018.1509707.Hepatitis.
3. Auriti C, De Rose DU, Santisi A, Martini L, Piersigilli F, Bersani I, Ronchetti MP, Caforio L. Pregnancy and viral infections: mechanisms of fetal damage, diagnosis and prevention of neonatal adverse outcomes from cytomegalovirus to SARS-CoV-2 and Zika virus. Biochim Biophys Acta Mol basis Dis. 2021;1867(10):166198. https://doi.org/10.1016/j.bbadis.2021.166198.
4. Baldo V, Baldovin T, Trivello R, Floreani A. Epidemiology of HCV infection. Curr Pharm Des. 2008;14:1646–54.
5. Castillo E, Murphy K, van Schalkwyk J. Hepatitis B and pregnancy. J Obstet Gynaecol Can.

2017;39:181–90. https://doi.org/10.1016/j.jogc.2016.11.001.
6. Lin CC, Hsieh HS, Huang YJ, et al. Hepatitis B virus infection among pregnant women in Taiwan: comparison between women born in Taiwan and other southeast countries. BMC Public Health. 2008;8:49. https://doi.org/10.1186/1471-2458-8-49.
7. Ding Y, Sheng Q, Ma L, et al. Chronic HBV infection among pregnant women and their infants in Shenyang, China. Virol J. 2013;10:17. https://doi.org/10.1186/1743-422X-10-17.
8. Bigna JJ, Kenne AM, Hamroun A, et al. Gender development and hepatitis B and C infections among pregnant women in Africa: a systematic review and meta-analysis. Infect Dis Poverty. 2019;8:16. https://doi.org/10.1186/s40249-019-0526-8.
9. Nelson NP, Jamieson DJ, Murphy TV. Prevention of perinatal hepatitis B virus transmission. J Pediatr Infect Dis Soc. 2014;3(Suppl 1):S7–12. https://doi.org/10.1093/jpids/piu064.
10. Tan J, Mao X, Zhang G, et al. Hepatitis B surface antigen positivity during pregnancy and risk of gestational diabetes mellitus: a systematic review and meta-analysis. J Viral Hepat. 2018;25(11):1372–83. https://doi.org/10.1111/jvh.12964.
11. Cui A-M, Shao J-G, Li H-B, et al. Association of chronic hepatitis B virus infection with preterm birth: our experience and meta-analysis. J Perinat Med. 2017;45:933–40. https://doi.org/10.1515/jpm-2016-0201.
12. Cui A-M, Cheng X-Y, Shao J-G, et al. Maternal hepatitis B virus carrier status and pregnancy outcomes: a prospective cohort study. BMC Pregnancy Childbirth. 2016;16:87. https://doi.org/10.1186/s12884-016-0884-1.
13. Wan Z, Zhou A, Zhu H, et al. Maternal hepatitis B virus infection and pregnancy outcomes: a hospital-based case-control study in Wuhan, China. J Clin Gastroenterol. 2018;52:73–8. https://doi.org/10.1097/MCG.0000000000000084.
14. Bartholomew ML, Lee M-J. Management of hepatitis B infection in pregnancy. Clin Obstet Gynecol. 2018;61:137–45. https://doi.org/10.1097/GRF.0000000000000331.
15. Le Campion A, Larouche A, Fauteux-Daniel S, Soudeyns H. Pathogenesis of hepatitis C during pregnancy and childhood. Viruses. 2012;4:3531–50.
16. Floreani A. Hepatitis C and pregnancy. World J Gastroenterol. 2013;19:6714. https://doi.org/10.3748/wjg.v19.i40.6714.
17. Pergam SA, Wang CC, Gardella CM, Sandison TG, Phipps WT, Hawes SE. Pregnancy complications associated with hepatitis C: data from a 2003-2005 Washington State Birth Cohort. Am J Obstet Gynecol. 2008;199:38.e1–9.
18. Connell LE, Salihu HM, Salemi JL, August EM, Weldeselasse H, Mbah AK. Maternal hepatitis B and hepatitis C carrier status and perinatal outcomes. Liver Int. 2011;31:1163–70.
19. Hurtado CW, Golden-Mason L, Brocato M, Krull M, Narkewicz MR, Rosen HR. Innate immune function in placenta and cord blood of hepatitis C-seropositive mother-infant dyads. PLoS One. 2010;5:e12232.
20. Seto MT, Cheung KW, Hung IFN. Management of viral hepatitis A, C, D and E in pregnancy. Best Pract Res Clin Obstet Gynaecol. 2020;68:44–53. https://doi.org/10.1016/j.bpobgyn.2020.03.009.
21. Benova L, Mohamoud YA, Clavert C, Abu-Raddad LJ. Vertical transmission of hepatitis C virus: systematic review and meta-analysis. Clin Infect Dis. 2014;59:765–73. https://doi.org/10.1093/cid/ciu447.
22. Roberts EA, Yeung L. Maternal-infant transmission of hepatitis C virus infection. Hepatology. 2002;36:S106–13.
23. European Paediatric Hepatitis C Virus Network. A significant sex—but not elective cesarean section—effect on mother-to-child transmission of hepatitis C virus infection. J Infect Dis. 2005;192:1872–9.
24. Pappalardo BL. Influence of maternal human immunodeficiency virus (HIV) co-infection on vertical transmission of hepatitis C virus (HCV): a meta-analysis. Int J Epidemiol. 2003;32:727–34.
25. Mast EE, Hwang LY, Seto DS, Nolte FS, Nainan OV, Wurtzel H, Alter MJ. Risk factors for perinatal transmission of hepatitis C virus (HCV) and the natural history of HCV infection acquired in infancy. J Infect Dis. 2005;192:1880–9.
26. Indolfi G, Resti M. Perinatal transmission of hepatitis C virus infection. J Med Virol. 2009;81:836–43.
27. England K, Thorne C, Newell ML. Vertically acquired paediatric coinfection with HIV and hepatitis C virus. Lancet Infect Dis. 2006;6:83–90.
28. Hayashida A, Inaba N, Oshima K, Nishikawa M, Shoda A, Hayashida S, Negishi M, Inaba F, Inaba M, Fukasawa I, et al. Re-evaluation of the true rate of hepatitis C virus mother-to-child transmission and its novel risk factors based on our two prospective studies. J Obstet Gynaecol Res. 2007;33:417–22.
29. Mavilia MG, Wu GY. Mechanisms and prevention of vertical transmission in chronic viral hepatitis. J Clin Transl Hepatol. 2017;5:119–29. https://doi.org/10.14218/JCTH.2016.00067.
30. Cryer AM, Imperial JC. Hepatitis B in pregnant women and their infants. Clin Liver Dis. 2019;23:451–62. https://doi.org/10.1016/j.cld.2019.04.007.
31. Cheung KW, Seto MTY, Lao TT-H. Prevention of perinatal hepatitis B virus transmission. Arch Gynecol Obstet. 2019;300:251–9. https://doi.org/10.1007/s00404-019-05190-0.
32. Liu J, Zhang S, Liu M, Wang Q, Shen H, Zhang Y. Maternal pre-pregnancy infection with hepatitis B virus and the risk of preterm birth: a population-based cohort study. Lancet Glob Health. 2017;5:e624–32. https://doi.org/10.1016/S2214-109X(17)30142-0.
33. Indolfi G, Easterbrook P, Dusheiko G, Siberry G, Chang M, Thorne C, et al. Hepatitis B virus infection in children and adolescents. Lancet Gastroenterol

Hepatol. 2019;4:466–76. https://doi.org/10.1016/S2468-1253(19)30042-1.
34. Giugliano S, Petroff MG, Warren BD, Jasti S, Linscheid C, Ward A, et al. Hepatitis C virus sensing by human trophoblasts induces innate immune responses and recruitment of maternal NK cells: potential implications for limiting vertical transmission. J Immunol. 2015;195:3737–47. https://doi.org/10.4049/jimmunol.1500409.
35. Piffer S, Mazza A, Dell'Anna L. Serological screening for hepatitis C during pregnancy: seroprevalence and maternal and neonatal outcomes in 45,000 pregnant women. Eur J Obstet Gynecol. 2020;254:195–9. https://doi.org/10.1016/j.ejogrb.2020.09.023.
36. Zinserling VA, Melnikova VF. Perinatal infections: questions of pathogenesis, morphological diagnostics and clinic-pathological correlations. Practical manual. SPb Elbi-SPb; 2002, 352p. (In Russian).
37. Douglas GC, Fazely F, Hu JJ. Transmission of HIV to the placenta, fetus and mother and implications of gametic infection. J Reprod Immunol. 1998;41(1–2):321–9.
38. Gaillard P, Verhofstede C, Mwanyumba F, Claeys P, et al. Exposure to HIV-1 during delivery and mother-to-child transmission. AIDS. 2000;14(15):2341–8.
39. Beima-Sofie KM, Bigham AW, Lingappa JR, Wamalwa D, et al. Toll-like receptor variants are associated with infant HIV-1 acquisition and peak plasma HIV-1 RNA level. AIDS. 2013;27(15):2431–9.
40. Tubiana R, Le Chenadec J, Rouzioux C, Mandelbrot L, et al. Factors associated with mother-to-child transmission of HIV-1 despite a maternal viral load <500 copies/ml at delivery: a case-control study nested in the French perinatal cohort (EPF-ANRS CO1). Clin Infect Dis. 2010;50(4):585–96.
41. Belyakov NA, Rakhmanina YN, Rakhmanova AG. Woman, child and HIV. SPb, Washington, BMEC; 2012, 600p. (In Russian).
42. Deblonde J, Claeys P, Temmerman M. Antenatal HIV screening in Europe: a review of policies. Eur J Public Health. 2007;17(5):414–8.
43. Drake AL, John-Stewart GC, Wald A, Mbori-Ngacha DA, et al. Herpes simplex virus type 2 and risk of intrapartum human immunodeficiency virus transmission. Obstet Gynecol. 2007;109(2 Pt 1):403–9.
44. Maiques V, García-Tejedor A, Perales A, Córdoba J, Esteban RJ. HIV detection in amniotic fluid samples. Amniocentesis can be performed in HIV pregnant women? Eur J Obstet Gynecol Reprod Biol. 2003;108(2):137–41.
45. Mohlala BK, Tucker TJ, Besser MJ, Williamson C, et al. Investigation of HIV in amniotic fluid from HIV-infected pregnant women at full term. J Infect Diss. 2005;192(3):488–91.
46. Viljoen J, Tuaillon E, Nagot N, Danaviah S, et al. Cytomegalovirus, and possibly Epstein-Barr virus, shedding in breast milk is associated with HIV-1 transmission by breastfeeding. AIDS. 2015;29(2):145–53.
47. Danaviah S, de Oliveira T, Bland R, Viljoen J, et al. Evidence of long-lived founder virus in mother-to-child HIV transmission. PLoS One. 2015;10(3):e0120389.
48. Johnson EL, Chakraborty R. HIV-1 at the placenta: immune correlates of protection and infection. Curr Opin Infect Dis. 2016;29(3):248–55.
49. Ross AL, Cannou C, Barré-Sinoussi F, Menu E. Proteasome-independent degradation of HIV-1 in naturally non-permissive human placental trophoblast cells. Retrovirology. 2009;6:46.
50. Marlin R, Nugeyre MT, de Truchis C, Berkane N, et al. Antigen-presenting cells represent targets for R5 HIV-1 infection in the first trimester pregnancy uterine mucosa. PLoS One. 2009;4:e5971.
51. Aebi-Popp K, Bailey H, Malyuta R, Volokha A, Thorne C. High prevalence of herpes simplex virus (HSV)-type 2 co-infection among HIV-positive women in Ukraine, but no increased HIV mother-to-child transmission risk. BMC Pregnancy Childbirth. 2016;16:94.
52. Fu C, Lu L, Wu H, Shaman J, et al. Placental antibody transfer efficiency and maternal levels: specific for measles, coxsackievirus A16, enterovirus 71, poliomyelitis I-III and HIV-1 antibodies. Sci Rep. 2016;6:38874.
53. Gumbo H, Chasekwa B, Church JA, Ntozini R, et al. Congenital and postnatal CMV and EBV acquisition in HIV-infected Zimbabwean infants. PLoS One. 2014;9(12):e114870.
54. Ocheke AN, Agaba PA, Imade GE, Silas OA, et al. Chorioamnionitis in pregnancy: a comparative study of HIV-positive and HIV-negative parturients. Int J STD AIDS. 2016;27(4):296–304.
55. Péré H, Rascanu A, LeGoff J, Matta M, et al. Herpes simplex virus type 2 (HSV-2) genital shedding in HSV-2-/HIV-1-co-infected women receiving effective combination antiretroviral therapy. Int J STD AIDS. 2016;27(3):178–85.
56. Singh L, Mishra S, Prasanna S, Cariappa MP. Seroprevalence of TORCH infections in antenatal and HIV positive patient populations. Med J Armed Forces India. 2015;71(2):135–8.
57. Kolobov AV, Merkulova AI, Zinserling VA. Infectious lesions of placenta as cause of miscarriage. J. Infectol. 2015;7(1):47–52. (In Russian).
58. Benirschke K, Burton GJ, Baergen RN. Pathology of the human placenta. 6th ed. Berlin: Springer; 2012, 941p.
59. Jauniaux E, Nessmann C, Imbert MC, Meuris S, et al. Morphological aspects of the placenta in HIV pregnancies. Placenta. 1988;9(6):633–42.
60. Jimenez E, Unger M, Vogel M, Lobeck H, et al. Morphologic studies of the placentas of HIV-positive mothers. Pathologe. 1988;9(4):228–34.
61. Martin AW, Brady K, Smith SI, DeCoste D, et al. Immunohistochemical localization of human immunodeficiency virus p24 antigen in placental tissue. Hum Pathol. 1992;23(4):411–4.

62. Backé E, Jiménez E, Unger M, Schäfer A, et al. Demonstration of HIV-1 infected cells in human placenta by in situ hybridisation and immunostaining. J Clin Pathol. 1992;45(10):871–4.
63. Katz JM, Fox CH, Eglinton GS, Meyers WA III, Queenan JT. Relationship between human immunodeficiency virus-1 RNA identification in placenta and perinatal transmission. J Perinatol. 1997;17(2):119–24.
64. Mwanyumba F, Gaillard P, Inion I, Verhofstede C, et al. Placental inflammation and perinatal transmission of HIV-1. J Acquir Immune Defic Syndr. 2002;29(3):262–9.
65. Vermaak A, Theron GB, Schubert PT, Kidd M, et al. Morphologic changes in the placentas of HIV-positive women and their association with degree of immune suppression. Int J Gynaecol Obstet. 2012;119(3):239–43.
66. Kriebs JM. Understanding herpes simplex virus: transmission, diagnosis, and considerations in pregnancy management. J Midwifery Womens Health. 2008;53:202–8. https://doi.org/10.1016/j.jmwh.2008.01.010.
67. Bradley H, Markowitz LE, Gibson T, McQuillan GM. Seroprevalence of herpes simplex virus types 1 and 2—United States, 1999–2010. J Infect Dis. 2014;209:325–33. https://doi.org/10.1093/infdis/jit458.
68. Pinninti SG, Kimberlin DW. Preventing herpes simplex virus in the newborn. Clin Perinatol. 2014;41:945–55. https://doi.org/10.1016/j.clp.2014.08.012.
69. Pinninti SG, Kimberlin DW. Neonatal herpes simplex virus infections. Semin Perinatol. 2018;42:168–75. https://doi.org/10.1053/j.semperi.2018.02.004.
70. Veal GJ, Errington J, Hayden J, Hobin D, Murphy D, Dommett RM, et al. Carboplatin therapeutic monitoring in preterm and full-term neonates. Eur J Cancer. 2015;51:2022–30. https://doi.org/10.1016/j.ejca.2015.07.011.
71. Shi T, Huang L, Xiong Y, Zhong Y, Yang J, Fu T, et al. The risk of Herpes Simplex Virus and human Cytomegalovirus infection during pregnancy upon adverse pregnancy outcomes: a meta-analysis. J Clin Virol. 2018;104:48–55. https://doi.org/10.1016/j.jcv.2018.04.016.
72. James SH, Kimberlin DW. Neonatal herpes simplex virus infection—epidemiology and treatment. Clin Perinatol. 2015;42:47–59. https://doi.org/10.1016/j.clp.2014.10.005.
73. Johnston C, Corey L. Current concepts for genital herpes simplex virus infection: diagnostics and pathogenesis of genital tract shedding. Clin Microbiol Rev. 2016;29:149–61. https://doi.org/10.1128/CMR.00043-15.
74. Akhtar J, Shukla D. Viral entry mechanisms: cellular and viral mediators of herpes simplex virus entry. FEBS J. 2009;276:7228–36. https://doi.org/10.1111/j.1742-4658.2009.07402.x.
75. Brown ZA, Wald A, Morrow RA, Selke S, Zeh J, Corey L. Effect of serologic status and cesarean delivery on transmission rates of herpes simplex virus from mother to infant. JAMA. 2003;289:203–9. https://doi.org/10.1001/jama.289.2.203.
76. Finger-Jardim F, Avila EC, Vanusa P, Gonçalves CV, de Martinez AMB, Soares MA. Prevalence of herpes simplex virus types 1 and 2 at maternal and fetal sides of the placenta in asymptomatic pregnant women. Am J Reprod Immunol. 2017;78:1–12. https://doi.org/10.1111/aji.12689.
77. Neuberger I, Garcia J, Meyers ML, Feygin T, Bulas DI, Mirsky DM. Imaging of congenital central nervous system infections. Pediatr Radiol. 2018;48:513–23.
78. Silasi M, Cardenas I, Racicot K, Kwon J-Y, Aldo P, Mor G. Viral infections during pregnancy. Am J Reprod Immunol. 2015;73:199–213. https://doi.org/10.1111/aji.12355.
79. Verevkina EV. Differentiated approach to the diagnosis and prevention of placental insufficiency in pregnant women with acute herpes virus infection. Chelyabinsk; 2009, 22p. (In Russian).
80. Milovanov AP, Serova OF, editors. Causes and differentiated treatment of early pregnancy loss (doctors manual). Moscow: Studio MDV; 2011, 216p. (In Russian).
81. Colugnati FA, Staras SA, Dollard SC, Cannon MJ. Incidence of cytomegalovirus infection among the general population and pregnant women in the United States. BMC Infect Dis. 2007;7:1–10. https://doi.org/10.1186/1471-2334-7-71.
82. Dreher AM, Arora N, Fowler KB, Novak Z, Britt WJ, Boppana SB, et al. Spectrum of disease and outcome in children with symptomatic congenital Cytomegalovirus infection. J Pediatr. 2014;164:855–9. https://doi.org/10.1016/j.jpeds.2013.12.007.Spectrum.
83. de Vries LS. Viral infections and the neonatal brain. Semin Pediatr Neurol. 2020;32:100769. https://doi.org/10.1016/j.spen.2019.08.005.
84. Naing ZW, Scott GM, Shand A, Hamilton ST, van Zuylen WJ, Basha J, et al. Congenital cytomegalovirus infection in pregnancy: a review of prevalence, clinical features, diagnosis and prevention. Aust N Z J Obstet Gynaecol. 2016;56:9–18. https://doi.org/10.1111/ajo.12408.
85. Lazzarotto T, Blázquez-Gamero D, Delforge M-L, Foulon I, et al. Congenital cytomegalovirus infection: a narrative review of the issues in screening and management from a panel of European experts. Front Pediatr. 2020;8:13.
86. van Zuylen WJ, Hamilton ST, Naing Z, Hall B, Shand A, Rawlinson WD. Congenital cytomegalovirus infection: clinical presentation, epidemiology, diagnosis and prevention. Obstet Med. 2014;7(4):140–6.
87. Walker SP, Palma-Dias R, Wood EM, Shekleton P, Giles ML. Cytomegalovirus in pregnancy: to screen or not to screen. BMC Pregnancy Childbirth. 2013;13:96.

88. Yamamoto AY, Castellucci RA, Aragon DC, Mussi-Pinhata MM. Early high CMV seroprevalence in pregnant women from a population with a high rate of congenital infection. Epidemiol Infect. 2013;141(10):2187–1291.
89. Mussi-Pinhata MM, Yamamoto AY, Moura Brito RM, et al. Birth prevalence and natural history of congenital cytomegalovirus infection in a highly seroimmune population. Clin Infect Dis. 2009;49(4):522–8.
90. Britt W. Controversies in the natural history of congenital human cytomegalovirus infection: the paradox of infection and disease in offspring of women with immunity prior to pregnancy. Med Microbiol Immunol. 2015;204:263–71. https://doi.org/10.1007/s00430-015-0399-9.
91. Britt WJ. Maternal immunity and the natural history of congenital human Cytomegalovirus infection. Viruses. 2018;10:405. https://doi.org/10.3390/v10080405.
92. Enders G, Daiminger A, Bäder U, Exler S, Enders M. Intrauterine transmission and clinical outcome of 248 pregnancies with primary cytomegalovirus infection in relation to gestational age. J Clin Virol. 2011;52:244–6. https://doi.org/10.1016/j.jcv.2011.07.005.
93. Kvitkina IG. Prevention and early diagnosis of placental insufficiency in pregnant women with herpes viral infection. Chelyabinsk; 2009, 19p. (In Russian).
94. Lim Y, Lyall H. Congenital cytomegalovirus—who, when, what-with and why to treat. J Inf Secur. 2017;74:S89–94. https://doi.org/10.1016/S0163-4453(17)30197-4.
95. Boppana SB, Fowler KB, Pass RF, Rivera LB, Bradford RD, Lakeman FD, et al. Congenital cytomegalovirus infection: association between virus burden in infancy and hearing loss. J Pediatr. 2005;146:817–23. https://doi.org/10.1016/j.jpeds.2005.01.059.
96. Christian LM, Iams JD, Porter K, Glaser R. Epstein-Barr virus reactivation during pregnancy and postpartum: effects of race and racial discrimination. Brain Behav Immun. 2012;26(8):1280–7. https://doi.org/10.1016/j.bbi.2012.08.006.
97. Kolobov A, Karev V. A case of intrauterine Epstein-Barr virus infection. Virchows Arch. 2017;471(Suppl. 1):S226.
98. Kim Y, Kim HS, Park JS, Kim CJ, Kim WH. Identification of Epstein-Barr virus in the human placenta and its pathologic characteristics. J Korean Med Sci. 2017;32(12):1959–66. https://doi.org/10.3346/jkms.2017.32.12.1959.
99. Ergaz Z, Ornoy A. Parvovirus B19 in pregnancy. Reprod Toxicol. 2006;21(4):421–35. https://doi.org/10.1016/j.reprotox.2005.01.006.
100. Pasquinelli G, Bonvicini F, Foroni L, Salfi N, Gallinella G. Placental endothelial cells can be productively infected by Parvovirus B19. J Clin Virol. 2009;44(3):3–38. https://doi.org/10.1016/j.jcv.2008.10.008.
101. Juhl D, Hennig H. Parvovirus B19: what is the relevance in transfusion medicine? Front Med (Lausanne). 2018;5:4. https://doi.org/10.3389/fmed.2018.00004.
102. Heegaard ED, Brown KE. Human Parvovirus B19. Clin Microbiol Rev. 2002;15(3):485–505. https://doi.org/10.1128/CMR.15.3.485-505.2002.
103. Pereira L. Congenital viral infection: traversing the uterine-placental Interface. Annu Rev Virol. 2018;5:273–99. https://doi.org/10.1146/annurev-virology-092917-043236.
104. Luo Y, Lou S, Deng X, Liu Z, Li Y, Kleiboeker S, et al. Parvovirus B19 infection of human primary erythroid progenitor cells triggers ATR-Chk1 signaling, which promotes B19 virus replication. J Virol. 2011;85:8046–55. https://doi.org/10.1128/JVI.00831-11.
105. Kolobov AV, Karev VE, Vorobtsova IN, Orel VI. Intrauterine infections with nonimmune hydrops fetalis. J Infectol. 2013;5(2):109–12. (In Russian).
106. Ornoy A, Ergaz Z. Parvovirus B19 infection during pregnancy and risks to the fetus. Birth Defects Res. 2017;109:311–23. https://doi.org/10.1002/bdra.23588.
107. Kolobov A, Karev V. A case of intrauterine parvovirus B19 infection. Virchows Arch. 2015;467(Suppl 1):S96.
108. Shi T, McAllister DA, O'Brien KL, et al. Global, regional, and national disease burden estimates of acute lower respiratory infections due to respiratory syncytial virus in young children in 2015: a systematic review and modelling study. Lancet. 2017;390:946–58.
109. Madhi SA, Cutland CL, Downs S, Jones S, van Niekerk N, Simoes EAF, Nunes MC. Burden of respiratory syncytial virus infection in South African human immunodeficiency virus (HIV)-infected and HIV-uninfected pregnant and postpartum women: a longitudinal cohort study. Clin Infect Dis. 2018;66(11):1658–65. https://doi.org/10.1093/cid/cix1088.
110. Stensballe LG, Ravn H, Kristensen K, Meakins T, Aaby P, Simoes EA. Seasonal variation of maternally derived respiratory syncytial virus antibodies and association with infant hospitalizations for respiratory syncytial virus. J Pediatr. 2009;154:296–8.
111. Roca A, Abacassamo F, Loscertales MP, et al. Prevalence of respiratory syncytial virus IgG antibodies in infants living in a rural area of Mozambique. J Med Virol. 2002;67:616–23.
112. Wheeler SM, Dotters-Katz S, Heine RP, Grotegut CA, Swamy GK. Maternal effects of respiratory syncytial virus infection during pregnancy. Emerg Infect Dis. 2015;21:1951–5.
113. Zinserling AV. Pecularities of lesions in viral and Mycoplasma infections of the respiratory tract. Virchows Arch A Pathol Pathol Anat. 1972;356(3):259–73.

114. Zinserling VA. Infectious pathology of the respiratory tract. Berlin: Springer; 2021. p. 36–7.
115. Kolobov AV, Karev VE. Viral placentitis: morphological features and verification possibilities. J Infect. 2018;10(4):24–9. (In Russian).
116. Mezouar S, Katsogiannou M, Amara AB, Bretelle F, Mege J-L. Placental macrophages: Origin, heterogeneity, function and role in pregnancy-associated infections. Placenta. 2021;103(103):94. https://doi.org/10.1016/j.placenta.2020.10.017.
117. Hosier H, Farhadian SF, Morotti RA, et al. SARS-CoV-2 infection of the placenta. J Clin Invest. 2020;130:4947–53. https://doi.org/10.1172/JCI139569.
118. Vivanti AJ, Vauloup-Fellous C, Prevot S, Zupan V, Suffee C, Do CJ, Benachi A, De Luca D. Transplacental transmission of SARS-CoV-2 infection. Nat Commun. 2020;11:3572. https://doi.org/10.1038/s41467-020-17436-6.
119. Facchetti F, Bugatti M, Drera E, Tripodo C, Sartori E, Cancila V, Papaccio M, Castellani R, Casola S, Boniotti MB, Cavadini P, Lavazza A. SARS-CoV2 vertical transmission with adverse effects on the newborn revealed through integrated immunohistochemical, electron microscopy and molecular analyses of placenta. EBioMedicine. 2020;59:102951. https://doi.org/10.1016/j.ebiom.2020.102951.
120. Schoenmakers S, Snijder P, Verdijk R, Kuiken T, Kamphuis S, Koopman L, Krasemann T, Rousian M, Broekhuizen M, Steegers E, Koopmans M, Fraaij P, Reiss I. SARS-CoV-2 placental infection and inflammation leading to fetal distress and neonatal multi-organ failure in an asymptomatic woman. J Pediatr Infect Dis. 2021;10:556.
121. Gesaka SR, Obimbo MM, Wanyoro A. Coronavirus disease 2019 and the placenta: a literature review. Placenta. 2022;126:209–23. https://doi.org/10.1016/j.placenta.2022.07.007.
122. Petrova VN, Russell CA. The evolution of seasonal influenza viruses [published correction appears in Nat Rev Microbiol. 2017 Nov 07]. Nat Rev Microbiol. 2018;16(1):47–60. https://doi.org/10.1038/nrmicro.2017.118.
123. Jamieson DJ, Honein MA, Rasmussen SA, et al. H1N1 2009 influenza virus infection during pregnancy in the USA. Lancet. 2009;374(9688):451–8. https://doi.org/10.1016/S0140-6736(09)61304-0.
124. Siston AM, Rasmussen SA, Honein MA, et al. Pandemic 2009 influenza A(H1N1) virus illness among pregnant women in the United States. JAMA. 2010;303(15):1517–25. https://doi.org/10.1001/jama.2010.479.
125. Neuzil KM, Reed GW, Mitchel EF, et al. Impact of influenza on acute cardiopulmonary hospitalizations in pregnant women. Am J Epidemiol. 1998;148(11):1094–102. https://doi.org/10.1093/oxfordjournals.aje.a009587.
126. Shu Y, Yu H, Li D. Lethal avian influenza A (H5N1) infection in a pregnant woman in Anhui Province, China. N Engl J Med. 2006;354(13):1421–2. https://doi.org/10.1056/NEJMc053524.
127. Gu J, Xie Z, Gao Z, et al. H5N1 infection of the respiratory tract and beyond: a molecular pathology study. Lancet. 2007;370(9593):1137–45. https://doi.org/10.1016/S0140-6736(07)61515-3.
128. Liong S, Oseghale O, To EE, et al. Influenza A virus causes maternal and fetal pathology via innate and adaptive vascular inflammation in mice. Proc Natl Acad Sci USA. 2020;117(40):24964–73. https://doi.org/10.1073/pnas.2006905117.
129. Al-Haddad B, Jacobsson B, Chabra S, et al. Long-term risk of neuropsychiatric disease after exposure to infection in utero. JAMA Psychiatry. 2019;76(6):594–602. https://doi.org/10.1001/jamapsychiatry.2019.0029.
130. Jacobsen H, Walendy-Gnirß K, Tekin-Bubenheim N, et al. Offspring born to influenza A virus infected pregnant mice have increased susceptibility to viral and bacterial infections in early life. Nat Commun. 2021;12(1):4957. https://doi.org/10.1038/s41467-021-25220-3.
131. Shuid AN, Jayusman PA, Shuid N, et al. Association between viral infections and risk of autistic disorder: an overview. Int J Environ Res Public Health. 2021;18(6):2817. https://doi.org/10.3390/ijerph18062817.
132. Lowe R, Barcellos C, Brasil P, et al. The Zika virus epidemic in Brazil: from discovery to future implications. Int J Environ Res Public Health. 2018;15(1):96. https://doi.org/10.3390/ijerph15010096.
133. Yu W, Hu X, Cao B. Viral infections during pregnancy: the big challenge threatening maternal and fetal health. Matern Fetal Med. 2022;4(1):72–86. https://doi.org/10.1097/FM9.0000000000000133.
134. Hcini N, Kugbe Y, Rafalimanana Z, et al. Association between confirmed congenital Zika infection at birth and outcomes up to 3 years of life. Nat Commun. 2021;12(1):3270. https://doi.org/10.1038/s41467-021-23468-3.
135. Britt WJ. Adverse outcomes of pregnancy-associated Zika virus infection. Semin Perinatol. 2018;42(3):155–67. https://doi.org/10.1053/j.semperi.2018.02.003.
136. Simoni MK, Jurado KA, Abrahams VM, et al. Zika virus infection of Hofbauer cells. Am J Reprod Immunol. 2017;77(2):e12613. https://doi.org/10.1111/aji.12613.
137. Tabata T, Petitt M, Puerta-Guardo H, et al. Zika virus targets different primary human placental cells, suggesting two routes for vertical transmission. Cell Host Microbe. 2016;20(2):155–66. https://doi.org/10.1016/j.chom.2016.07.002.
138. Wells MF, Salick MR, Wiskow O, et al. Genetic ablation of AXL does not protect human neural progenitor cells and cerebral organoids from Zika virus infection. Cell Stem Cell. 2016;19(6):703–8. https://doi.org/10.1016/j.stem.2016.11.011.
139. Hastings AK, Yockey LJ, Jagger BW, et al. TAM receptors are not required for Zika virus infection

in mice. Cell Rep. 2017;19(3):558–68. https://doi.org/10.1016/j.celrep.2017.03.058.

140. Bayer A, Lennemann NJ, Ouyang Y, Bramley JC, Morosky S, Marques ETDA, Cherry S, Sadovsky Y, Coyne CB. Type III interferons produced by human placental trophoblasts confer protection against Zika virus infection. Cell Host Microbe. 2016;19:705–12. https://doi.org/10.1016/j.chom.2016.03.008.
141. Wang Y, Zhao S. Vascular biology of the placenta. San Rafael: Morgan & Claypool Life Sciences; 2010. http://www.ncbi.nlm.nih.gov/books/NBK53247/. PMID: 21452443.
142. de Noronha L, Zanluca C, Azevedo MLV, Luz KG, Santos CNDD. Zika virus damages the human placental barrier and presents marked fetal neurotropism. Mem Inst Oswaldo Cruz. 2016;111:287–93. https://doi.org/10.1590/0074-02760160085.
143. Jurado KA, Simoni MK, Tang Z, Uraki R, Hwang J, Householder S, Wu M, Lindenbach BD, Abrahams VM, Guller S, Fikrig E. Zika virus productively infects primary human placenta-specific macrophages. JCI Insight. 2016;1:e88461. https://doi.org/10.1172/jci.insight.88461.
144. Adibi JJ, Zhao Y, Cartus AR, Gupta P, Davidson LA. Placental mechanics in the zika-microcephaly relationship. Cell Host Microbe. 2016;20:9–11. https://doi.org/10.1016/j.chom.2016.06.013.
145. Zimmerman MG, Quicke KM, O'Neal JT, Arora N, Machiah D, Priyamvada L, Kauffman RC, Register E, Adekunle O, Swieboda D, Johnson EL, Cordes S, Haddad L, Chakraborty R, Coyne CB, Wrammert J, Suthar MS. Cross-reactive dengue virus antibodies augment Zika virus infection of human placental macrophages. Cell Host Microbe. 2018;24:731–742.e6. https://doi.org/10.1016/j.chom.2018.10.008.
146. Quicke KM, Bowen JR, Johnson EL, McDonald CE, Ma H, O'Neal JT, Rajakumar A, Wrammert J, Rimawi BH, Pulendran B, Schinazi RF, Chakraborty R, Suthar MS. Zika virus infects human placental macrophages. Cell Host Microbe. 2016;20:83–90. https://doi.org/10.1016/j.chom.2016.05.015.
147. Gavegnano C, Bassit LC, Cox BD, Hsiao H-M, Johnson EL, Suthar M, Chakraborty R, Schinazi RF. Jak inhibitors modulate production of replication-competent Zika virus in human Hofbauer, trophoblasts, and neuroblastoma cells. Pathog Immun. 2017;2:199–218. https://doi.org/10.20411/pai.v2i2.190.

7 Transplacental Transmission Infections: Infections Due to Mycoplasma and Protozoa

7.1 Mycoplasmosis

Mycoplasmas is a separate class of Mollicutes pathogens characterized by the absence of a rigid cell wall, pronounced polymorphism, and the ability to reproduce by forming particles whose size does not exceed 200 nm. Most of the 40 species of the Mycoplasmataceae family belong to the genus Mycoplasma; in addition, the genus Ureaplasma has been isolated, the typical representative of which is *U. urealyticum*. Mycoplasma infections of various localizations are quite widespread in humans and many animals. It should be noted that they often occur latently, which makes their diagnosis difficult. Changes in the lungs, brain, and other organs characteristic of mycoplasmosis have been described in numerous studies of the Zinserling's scientific school [1–4].

A very important role of these pathogens in the unfavorable course of pregnancy, which is accompanied by severe complications for the woman and fetus, has been revealed. In addition, this infection is responsible for a significant part of stillbirths, premature births, and the birth of sick children.

Widespread study of mycoplasmoses began in the early 1960s, since R. M. Chanock et al. (1962) showed the pathogenicity of mycoplasmas (Eaton's agent, PPLO factor). In 1965, Driscoll was the first to point out the connection between mycoplasma secretion and spontaneous abortions. Somewhat later, similar results were obtained in the works of C. Alexandre et al. (1967); H.J. Harwich (1967). These researchers isolated the pathogens of *M. hominis* and T-mycoplasma from couples where pregnancy ended with spontaneous abortions. An increase in antibody titers was also detected. It has now been established that the relatively recently discovered pathogen of urogenital mycoplasmosis, *M. genitalium*, has a significant antigenic affinity with M. pneumoniae and therefore they can overlap during immunofluorescence examination and in serological reactions. It is also important that mycoplasmas of various types can be isolated from the organs of fetuses and newborns.

The disadvantage of many studies is the lack of a morphological description of the lesion of the afterbirth. The first description was made by D. M. Jones. The author studied the afterbirth of 62 spontaneous miscarriages and found fields of leukocyte infiltration in the septa, around the large vessels of the chorial plate and umbilical cord vessels. Necrotic foci and polymorphonuclear leukocytes were also detected in the basal lamina. Similar changes were found in the amnion. Among the works of a later period, there are only a few descriptions of the morphological picture of mycoplasma placentitis, usually caused by *M. hominis* in cases of miscarriages or fetuses and children who died in the perinatal period due to ascending infection. There is also an opinion about possible infection from the appendages of the uterus or hematogenically. This point of view

V. Zinserling et al., *Placentitis and Perinatal Infections*,
https://doi.org/10.1007/978-3-031-80553-0_7

is also confirmed by the fact that placentitis can be found in the afterbirth during cesarean delivery. It should be noted that there are few works on mycoplasmosis in the literature of recent years.

The most complete information about ultrastructural changes in the placenta in mycoplasmosis is provided by N.R. Shabunina et al. Mycoplasmas of typical structure were detected by them in the interstitial space. They looked like ellipsoid formations surrounded by a membrane with flake-like contents inside. Their appearance corresponded to the appearance of mycoplasmas obtained from culture media and studied by EM. There were two variants of syncytiotrophoblast cells. The first of them was represented by hyperchromic cells with a large number of ribosomes and polysomes and a well-developed granular endoplasmic network. There are a lot of mitochondria in the cytoplasm. A granular-looking mitochondrial matrix with single crystals, organelles with a complete absence of crystals were identified. Lysosomes and autophagosomes were found in the cells as well as membrane structures resembling myelin-like formations. The nuclei of such cells are hyperchromic, lobed nuclei with uneven chromatin distribution were observed. Another type of cells was represented by light cells with the absence of villi or their sharp decrease. In cells of this type, a sharp decrease in ribosomes and polysomes was observed. The tubules and cisterns of the endoplasmic reticulum are sharply expanded, and they formed rather large vacuoles with fine-grained contents. Single ribosomes were preserved on the membranes of the granular endoplasmic reticulum. There are many "empty" mitochondria in the cytoplasm with a violation of the double-contour of the membranes and a complete absence of crists. In some of them, fine-grained matrix and fragments of crists were visible. "Membrane" formations were observed in single mitochondria. Lysosomes were found in the cytoplasm of such cells, and bundles of fibrils were found in the cytoplasmic matrix.

The basal layer of the fruit capillaries is uneven: loosened, thickened, or thinned in places. The endothelium of medium electron density bulges out into the lumen. Fibrils, single mitochondria with a granular matrix and single crystals are found in the cytoplasm. The nuclei have an uneven distribution of chromatin.

We present the results of a study of previous years conducted jointly with V.F. Melnikova. A total of 62 placentas with mycoplasma lesions were specially studied in detail. Of these, 21 cases were monoinfection and 41 mixed.

Macroscopically, the placenta was not significantly altered. Irregular or triangular white areas with a dense consistency were detected in the tissue (four cases), foci of old and fresh hemorrhages (three times) and foci of softening, sometimes filled with serous or jelly-like contents. These plots, however, did not occupy a significant amount (up to 5–7%). The membranes of the afterbirth in most cases were smooth, thin, and in two afterbirths, they were diffusely thickened at the distal edge of the fetal sac and in two more they had multiple plaque-like thickenings. The umbilical cord was correctly developed in all cases, and changes in decidual cells and peripheral trophoblast characteristic of mycoplasma infection are detected in the basal plates and septa of placentas of this group. Later on, such cells undergo balloon alteration, the nuclei become pyknotic and necrotize. When PAS sections are stained, pas-positive inclusions (mycoplasmas) are detected in vacuoles. They are also determined when stained with azur-eosin in the form of azurophilic grains.

The vascular endothelium is exfoliated in places. The walls of the vessels are significantly thickened and homogenized. Multiple lymphocytic infiltrates are constantly found in the basal lamina with an admixture of neutrophilic leukocytes and plasmocytes. Foci of predominantly colliquational necrosis and cysts were also detected.

Similar changes are defined in the septs. There is a characteristic transformation of decidual cells with subsequent vacuolization and colliquation necrosis, sometimes cysts with serous contents are detected.

In all studied placentas of this group, there is a focal or disseminated lesion of the villous chorion with the involvement of villi of different caliber in the infectious process. The most significant changes occur in the anchor, intermediate and terminal villi. They consist primarily in the defeat of the syncytiotrophoblast and cytotrophoblast of the villi, which becomes thickened, and its cytoplasm is light, foamy. Characteristic changes also occur in the stroma of the villi during mycoplasma infection. Part of the villi contains light cells with extensive foamy cytoplasm, in which pas-positive corpuscles are detected. Langhans cells undergo a similar transformation. At the same time, there is a significant increase in the size of the villi, narrowing of the interstitial spaces.

In some cases, lymphocytic infiltrates are detected in the stroma of the villi (usually in the anchored or located near the basal plate). In the interstitial space, there are quite constantly small accumulations of lymphoid elements with an admixture of leukocytes.

With destructive changes in the trophoblast of the villi, fibrin is deposited, in which the villi are walled up. They show necrobiotic changes with homogenization of the villi stroma and pyknosis of the nuclei. Macroscopically, these areas look like white infarcts.

Prolonged damage to the placenta involving the villous chorion leads to stroma fibrosis and villous deformation. In addition, there is a significant proliferation of stroma cells, thickening of the vessel walls and significant narrowing, as well as obliteration of the lumens with reduction of the vascular bed. These changes are noted in both small vessels and large vessels of stem villi.

When the placenta is affected by mycoplasmas, changes occur in the amnion similar to those described in other organ structures. Lesions are detected in the chorial plate as well. Vacuolization of the peripheral trophoblast and pyknosis of the nuclei are also noted. In some cases, lymphoid infiltrates with an admixture of leukocytes are found in it. As a rule, they are located along the edge of the placental disc (Fig. 7.1).

The extraplacental membranes of the afterbirth are also significantly altered during microscopic examination. The nature of the changes in the extraplacental membranes is similar to those observed in other organ structures.

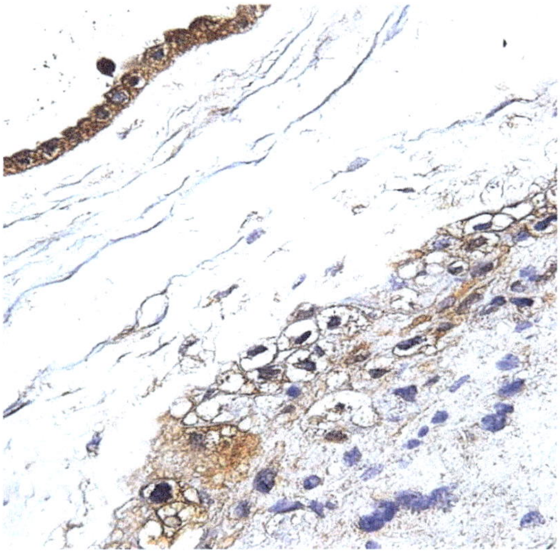

Fig. 7.1 Placentitis in mycoplasma infection IHC ×200

Currently, we have also studied the morphological manifestations of lesions of the afterbirth caused by ureaplasmas. The only human pathogen belonging to this genus of the Mycoplasmataceae family is *Ureaplasma urealyticum*. It is characterized by the need for growth in urea and small delicate colonies, which led to its former name T-strains (from the English tiny—gentle). There is quite a large clinical and microbiological literature characterizing the ability of this pathogen to cause a variety of inflammatory processes in the genital and urinary organs, although the possibility of asymptomatic carriage is also reported. There is practically no data on the nature of structural changes.

According to our observations, inflammatory changes in ureaplasmosis can be detected in all parts of the afterbirth, but the most characteristic for it are lesions of the extraplacental membranes and basal lamina. The similarity of changes caused by ureaplasmas and mycoplasmas is noted. The characteristic localization of the pathogen in the severe manifest forms of the disease studied by us is intracellular. In the affected cells, vacuolization of mainly peripheral sections of the cytoplasm is noted, and later its lysis, often in the form of rather large foci. Cyst-like cavities appear at the site of colliquation necrosis. Weakly or moderately pronounced lymphocytic-macrophage-neutrophil infiltration is noted in the affected areas. In the villous chorion, there is an increase in small anchor villi with the opening of stromal channels, vacuolization of stroma cells. Unlike mycoplasmosis, vascular wall changes are less pronounced.

Thus, the conducted study showed a fairly significant frequency of mycoplasmic etiology placentas, which have well-defined morphological manifestations. It was noted that they are very similar when infected with mycoplasmas of different types. In several modern publications the role of mycoplasma and ureaplasma in perinatal pathology is confirmed, but no data on pathology are presented [5, 6].

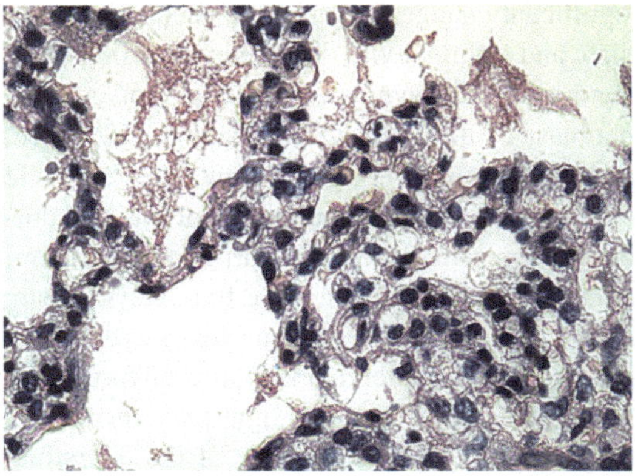

Fig. 7.2 Lung lesions in intrauterine mycoplasma infection. Note vacuolization of enlarged cells. H-E ×200

7.1.1 Intrauterine Mycoplasmosis

The ability of mycoplasmas to cause intrauterine infection was shown in the descriptions of single observations in the late 1960s and early 1970s of the twentieth century. The most complete information about intrauterine mycoplasmosis was obtained in Russia in the 1970s by various teams in Leningrad (A.V. Zinserling et al.), Moscow (B.S. Guzman et al.), Chisinau (I.G. Schroit, A.S. Kozlyuk) as a result of studying a variety of autopsy and experimental materials [1–4].

Unfortunately, in the future, due to a number of objective and subjective reasons, researchers began to pay less attention to this pathology. At the same time, our data allow us to talk about the preservation of this infection of an important role in the etiology of intrauterine infections at the present time.

The issue of the location of mycoplasmas is currently being discussed. Many authors consider mycoplasmas as an extracellular pathogen located on the surface of cell membranes. In numerous studies, including those performed with the help of EM, within the framework of our scientific school, the ability of mycoplasmas to both intracellular (in the most severe course of the disease) and extracellular location (in mild forms) has been repeatedly proven [3, 4]. According to our data, the most characteristic feature of intrauterine mycoplasmosis is the reproduction of mycoplasmas in epithelial cells. Changes in alveolocytes are especially typical in the respiratory organs, along with this, protein masses, erythrocytes and sometimes a small number of granular leukocytes are found in the lumen of the alveoli and small bronchi (Fig. 7.2). Circulatory disorders are also noted in the form of increased blood filling of vessels of all calibers, hemorrhages in the alveoli and sometimes thrombosis of blood vessels. Moderate lymphohistiocytic infiltration is often detected, as well as fibrosis of the peribronchial and, to a lesser extent, perivascular and interalveolar interstitial tissue. Macroscopic changes are moderate and non-specific.

Pronounced changes are found in the liver. With light microscopy, mycoplasmas can be detected in the cytoplasm of some hepatocytes and Kupffer cells. These cells undergo alterative changes, vacuoles naturally appear in hepatocytes that do not contain either fat or glycogen. Along with this, hyperplasia of Kupffer cells, discomplexation of hepatic beams, stagnant fullness, and expansion of the sinusoidal spaces are revealed. The expansion of the bile capillaries naturally occurs with the accumulation of bile in them, despite the fact that the bile ducts are not dilated and their patency is preserved. Lymphohistiocytic infiltration is noted around the bile ducts. Kidney changes are of great interest. For the first time, W. Pachas (1970) mentioned the possibility of developing renal cell damage in this disease. The works of our scientific school show changes in the epithelium of mainly distal sections of the nephron, where mycoplasma reproduction is primarily observed. As a result, there is a gradually increasing vacuolization of the nephrothelium. Later on, necrotic changes occur, followed by the rejection of dead cells. Protein masses accumulate in the lumen of the tubules, individual neutrophilic leukocytes, and sometimes numerous erythrocytes appear, hyaline and granular cylinders are found in some places. With a significant duration of the disease, regeneration of the tubular epithelium is detected. There is also some restructuring of the organ. Glomeruli are often enlarged in size, their loops are swollen, unevenly full-blooded. The mesangial skeleton is expanded due to the accumulation of pas-positive material in it and focal cell proliferation. Protein rich fluid, several desquamated epithelial cells of the capsule and sometimes single erythrocytes accumulate in the capsules of the renal bodies. The interstitial tissue of the kidneys, especially in the medulla, is edematous, rich in acidic mucopolysaccharides. Blood vessels are dilated, their endothelium is often swollen and partially desquamated.

There may also be a lesion in the intestine caused by mycoplasmas. It consists primarily in an epithelial lesion similar to the one described above in the lungs. Endotheliocytes and ganglion cells of intramural nodes of the autonomic nervous system can undergo similar changes. In its own plate of the mucous membrane, there is fullness, edema, small hemorrhages and rather thick lymphoplasmocytic infiltrates with an admixture of individual neutrophilic leukocytes.

In the brain, studied in the most detail by V.A. Zinserling years ago, histological examination shows fullness of the soft meninges, an increase in the number of macrophage cells in them. The vacuolized cytoplasm of many of them contains mycoplasmas. There is no clear stratification in the cerebral cortex, and poorly differentiated elements predominate among their cells. Many neurons of the cortex, as well as the nodes of the base, turn pale and undergo a metamorphosis characteristic of mycoplasmosis. Nerve cells with "ischemic" changes are also identified. However, there is no pronounced glial reaction. Ependymocytes are often incorrectly oriented, and mycoplasmas are present in the cytoplasm of some of them. Similar changes are naturally detected in the cells of the lining of the choroidal plexuses. Clusters of poorly differentiated glial elements may be observed around the ventricular system.

Macroscopically, swelling and fullness of the soft meninges, flabbiness of the brain matter are detected, and small hemorrhages may also occur. Fundamentally similar metamorphosis, in addition to non-specific changes, can be detected from part of the cells of more deeply located areas of the definitive cortex and in the fetal adrenal cortex.

In intrauterine mycoplasmosis, lesions of other organs and tissues, including the cardiovascular system, are also observed. The changes characteristic of mycoplasmosis with the presence of mycoplasmas in cardiomyocytes, endothelium of the endocardium and intracardiac vessels, as well as the occurrence of metamorphosis of affected cells, are described. Along with this, there are also non-specific processes in the form of microcirculation disorders and alterative changes in cardiomyocytes. With a prolonged course of the disease or in combination with other infectious diseases, disorganization of the connective tissue of the endocardium and myocardium may develop in the form of mucoid and fibrinoid swelling, perivascular lymphohistiocytic infiltrates and productive vasculitis occur.

When examining the lymphoid system in intrauterine mycoplasmosis in children, hyperplasia of reticuloepitheliocytes of the thymus gland, reticular cells of the spleen and lymph nodules, endotheliocytes of the sinuses of lymph nodes, as well as endotheliocytes of blood vessels of the same organs was revealed. Mycoplasmas were detected in the affected cells, in the area of which vacuolization of the cytoplasm was noted. The endotheliocytes of the sinuses were partially desquamated. Along with this, non-specific changes were also detected—accidental involution of the thymus gland of varying severity. Lymphoblasts, usually in small quantities, as well as macrophages and sometimes single hematopoietic cells appeared in the cerebral cords of the paracortical zone and the red pulp of the spleen. There were also signs of premature maturation of the lymphoid system. It should be noted that the localization of these changes was different in different observations and depended on the pathways of mycoplasma dissemination, among which hematogenic prevailed, but lymphogenic spread of infection was also noted. This was especially clearly revealed when the process was localized in the lungs, in which bronchopulmonary lymph nodes are quite naturally affected.

It should be specially noted that these changes can develop even antenatally, since they are also detected in stillbirths. The fundamental similarity of lesions caused by different types of mycoplasmas in late miscarriages (with a weight of 300–900 g) with those described above is shown.

Of great interest are the data of P.M. Mitrofanov, who managed to give a detailed morphological characterization of intrauterine mycoplasmosis in calves, both during spontaneous abortions and experimental infection of cows. The changes he identified were very similar to those described by us in deceased children and fetuses [3].

7.2 Toxoplasmosis

In the countries with the moderate climate, the only relative frequent perinatal infection of protozoal origin is toxoplasmosis. This disease has been studied most fully in the middle of twentieth century [7–11]. In the recent publications [12], the older data have been confirmed. It has been established that with the latent form of toxoplasmosis in a pregnant woman, infection of the afterbirth can occur from the source of infection in the endometrium. The possibility of hematogenous infection of the afterbirth in the acute form of toxoplasmosis in a pregnant woman is not excluded. It has been shown that macroscopically, the placenta in toxoplasmosis can be unchanged or enlarged, pale, and resembles the placenta in the edematous form of hemolytic disease. Chronic sluggish villitis was described, in which focal disseminated villi lesion was noted. In the stroma of the villi, predominant lymphoid infiltration with an admixture of plasma cells, an increase in Hofbauer cells, fibrosis and sometimes foci of necrosis are revealed. W.G. Elliott (1970) described granulomas in the villi and noted the development of endarteritis, as well as clusters of monocytes in the interstitial spaces. G. Altschuller (1973) identifies an edematous form of placental toxoplasmosis, in which in the stroma of the villi, a large number of Hofbauer cells are noted, and pathogens are also detected in the villi. Toxoplasma placentitis can lead to miscarriage, stillbirth, or fetal infection. Histological examination reveals chronic villusitis, in which groups of villi are affected. In their stroma, lymphoid infiltration is detected with an admixture of plasmocytes, macrophages, and sometimes granulomas are formed. Clusters of lymphocytes and macrophages are found in the intervillous space. The lesion of villous vessels with the development of vasculitis is characteristic. Pathognomonic for toxoplasmosis is the detection of the pathogen lying freely or in the form of pseudocysts.

The manifestations of toxoplasmosis in newborns at the early stages of development are generalized. At this time, small areas of necrosis appear in all affected organs in the locations of toxoplasmas. Here, more common infiltrates are visible in the interstitial tissue, consisting of lymphocytes, histiocytes, as well as plasmocytes, neutrophilic, and eosinophilic leukocytes.

Liver damage is most often described. It is interstitial hepatitis with small areas of necrosis and pronounced peri-portal infiltration, followed later by fibrosis. Along with this, extramedullary hematopoiesis is revealed. The spleen is hyperplastic, and moderate infiltration by eosinophilic leukocytes is possible. In the myocardium, respiratory organs, adrenal glands and, less often, in other internal organs, small areas of necrosis and infiltration of interstitial tissue are noted. Similar focal changes occur in the brain and eyes, but they do not play a leading role during this period of toxoplasmosis. An exanthema is typical, having the character of a roseolous or macular papular rash.

In the later stages of intrauterine toxoplasmosis—a few months or years after birth—brain

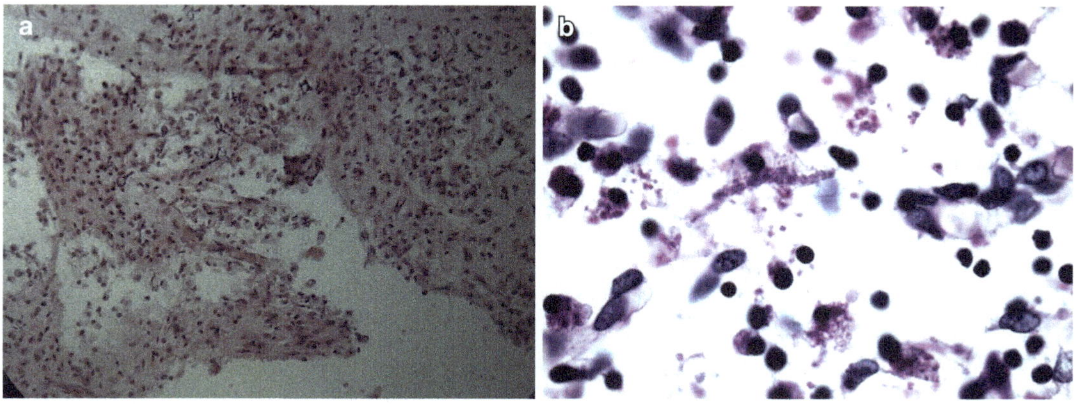

Fig. 7.3 Formation of brain cyst. (**a**) H-E, ×100, (**b**) numerous toxoplasma. PAS-reaction ×600

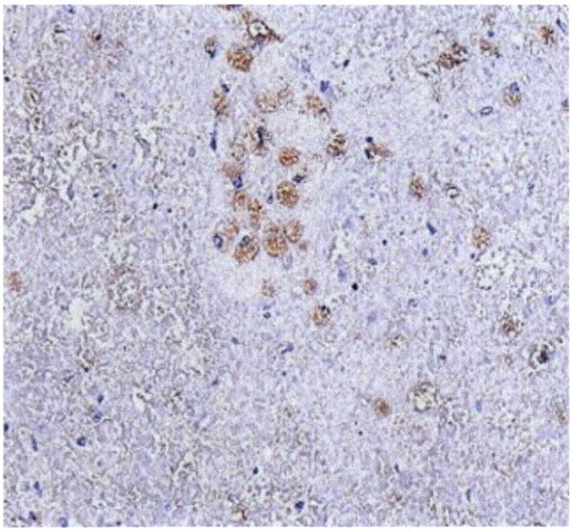

Fig. 7.4 Toxoplasma in brain tissue. IHC ×200

damage is sharply predominant. Toxoplasmas are found in its substance both in nerve cells and extracellularly (Figs. 7.3 and 7.4). Dystrophic and then necrotic changes occur. The exudative reaction, especially the leukocyte reaction, is very poorly expressed. Instead, a macrophage reaction is observed. Macrophages, mainly of glial origin, phagocytize pathogens, and decay products of necrotized brain tissue. Stasis, swelling of the endothelium, proliferation of adventitia cells, and often thrombosis are noted in the blood vessels. As a result of vascular damage, secondary focal aseptic colliquation necrosis of brain tissue occurs .

Necrosis foci are located asymmetrically, mainly in the cortex of the cerebral hemispheres and in the subependimar zone of the lateral ventricles in both the gray and white matter. They can vary dramatically in their size and number. With the greatest severity of the process, these foci merge together into continuous yellowish stripes running along the convolutions of the cerebral cortex. Ependymal defects may be detected on the walls of the ventricles. The nasal plexuses and meninges are often thickened, whitish or yellowish in color.

Later on, the necrotic tissue resolves with the formation of cysts. They are especially often located on the border between the gray and white matter of the large hemispheres. Cerebrospinal fluid is located in the cavities, and macrophages containing decay products of brain tissue in the cytoplasm are found on their walls. The necrosis sites are delimited by glial growths, as a result of which the brain substance surrounding the cysts turns out to be devoid of the usual structure and sharply compacted. Vascular plexuses and soft cerebral membranes are also subjected to adhesion. Due to impaired cerebrospinal fluid outflow, internal dropsy of the brain develops. In parallel, there is an association with pulverized or granular, and sometimes massive lime deposits. Calcification is not specific to toxoplasmosis; therefore, it cannot be diagnosed on the basis of a single focal calcification.

At the same stage of toxoplasmosis, eye changes can also be detected—chorioretinitis, manifested in focal infiltration of the membranes of the eyes and the development of small areas of necrosis. This leads to a thickening of the retina and vascular membrane. Other areas of the eye are less often affected. Later, granulation tissue develops here and synechiae are formed.

Sometimes skin lesions are possible. Superficial and deep perivascular infiltrates are detected on the trunk, consisting mainly of lymphocytes and histiocytes as well as macrophages, plasmocytes, and eosinophils. In addition, hemorrhages and sometimes allergic vasculitis are noted. Calcification, sometimes diffuse, of the upper layers of the skin is also possible. Macroscopically, the foci have the character of papulo-hemorrhagic, papulo-nodular, and infiltrative necrotic elements.

Intrauterine toxoplasmosis is often accompanied by impaired brain development, expressed to varying degrees. Underdevelopment of one lobe and even the entire cerebral hemispheres can be observed. There are descriptions of the association with toxoplasmosis of other malformations.

References

1. Zinserling (Tsinzerling) AV, Avtushenko SS, Vydumkina SP, et al. Intrauterine infection caused by Myc. hominis. Probl Matern Child Care. 1982;27(7):32–4. (In Russian).
2. Zinserling (Tsinzerling) AV, Vydumkina SP. About the frequency of intrauterine infections caused by respiratory viruses, Mycoplasma hominis and role of serological study in their diagnosis. Arkh Patol. 1982;44(1):24–9. (In Russian).
3. Zinserling AV, Zinserling VA. Modern infections: pathologic anatomy and issues of pathogenesis: a guide. SPb: Sotis; 2002, 346p. (In Russian).
4. Zinserling VA. School of infectious pathology of A.V. Zinserling: achievements and perspectives. Arkh Patol. 2014;76(1):3–9. (In Russian).
5. Noda-Nicolau NM, Tantengco OAG, Polettini J, et al. Genital mycoplasmas and biomarkers of inflammation and their association with spontaneous preterm birth and preterm prelabor rupture of membranes: a systematic review and meta-analysis. Front Microbiol. 2022;13:859732. https://doi.org/10.3389/fmicb.2022.859732.
6. Matasariu DR, Ursache A, Agache A, et al. Genital infection with *Ureaplasma urealyticum* and its effect on pregnancy. Exp Ther Med. 2022;23:89. https://doi.org/10.3892/etm.2021.11012.
7. Procop GW, Pritt BS, editors. Pathology of infectious diseases. Amsterdam: Elsevier; 2015, 706p.
8. Hofman P. Infectious disease and parasites. Berlin: Springer; 2016, 343p.
9. Herrington CS. Muir's textbook of pathology. Boca Raton: CRC Press; 2020. ISBN 9780367146726.
10. Zinserling AV, Zinserling VA. Modern infections: pathologic anatomy and issues of pathogenesis: a guide. SPb: Sotis. 2002, 346p. (In Russian).
11. Kradin RL. Diagnostic pathology of infectious diseases. Amsterdam: Elsevier; 2018, 698p.
12. Arranz-Solís D, Mukhopadhyay D, Saeij JJP. Toxoplasma effectors that affect pregnancy outcome. Trends Parasitol. 2021;37(4):283–95. https://doi.org/10.1016/j.pt.2020.10.013.

8 Role of Biological Pathogens in Malformations

Birth defects are the leading cause of infant death, accounting for 20% of all infant deaths, so preventing birth defects is an important social goal [1]. Yet, the etiology of birth defects is complex, which means that there are many pathways for improvement. Modern teratology pays special attention to genetic studies in order to reveal certain gene and chromosome pathology. In sporadic malformations, it is usually impossible to detect stable gene defect in all cases. But even in genetic not inherited syndromes with clarified pathogenesis, the primary course of their development remains unclear. Taking in consideration that many intracellular microorganisms being in dormant state and lied with different structures including DNA, we may propose that the real role of pathogens may be underestimated.

Several types of viral infections during pregnancy have been clarified to contribute the higher risks of congenital abnormalities, such as Zika virus, rubella, and hepatitis B virus [2–5].

ZIKV is spread globally from 2015 to 2016 and led to a Public Health Emergency of International Concern declared by the WHO due to emerging neuropathogenicity such as the Guillain–Barré syndrome in adults and microcephaly in neonates, respectively [6]. Moreover, the fetal congenital Zika syndrome (CZS), a unique pattern of birth defects and disabilities found among fetuses and babies born to mothers exposed to ZIKV during pregnancy, has attracted extensive attention since the most recent epidemics in the Americas [7].

Until now, >4000 infants worldwide have laboratory-confirmed CZS [6, 8]. A study of Brazilian infants with microcephaly caused by ZIKV infection revealed that 93% of infants had brain calcification, 69% encountered cortical developmental malformations such as lissencephaly and pachygyria, and 66% developed ventriculomegaly due to brain atrophy [9]. Following studies have demonstrated that 35–70% of infants with microcephaly and cerebral calcification are accompanied by a spectrum of ocular alterations such as optic nerve hypoplasia and double-ring sign, foveal reflex loss, chorioretinal macular atrophy, and cataracts [10].

Mechanistically, Li et al. reported a direct link between ZIKV infection in the embryonic brain and microcephaly by disrupting neural progenitor development in a mouse model, which could provide valuable resources for further exploration of the underlying mechanisms and management of ZIKV-related pathological effects [11]. Besides the above-mentioned disorders, musculoskeletal, genitourinary, and pulmonary abnormalities are also observed in CZS babies, indicating phenotypic diversity caused by congenital ZIKV infection [12–14]. Sadly, up to now, very little is understood about the pathogenic mechanisms underlying the vertical transmission of ZIKV. It has been reported that ZIKV can infect human and mouse blastocysts in vitro,

V. Zinserling et al., *Placentitis and Perinatal Infections*,
https://doi.org/10.1007/978-3-031-80553-0_8

especially in trophectoderm which gives rise to various trophoblast lineages in the mature placenta. This result indicates that ZIKV infection may directly lead to the developmental restriction of blastocysts and trophoblast stem cells through apoptosis and necrosis pathway, and eventually cause the occurrence of severe CZS [15]. However, whether ZIKV could infect blastocysts and induce any embryonic abnormality in vivo remains unknown. If it is true, it could explain at least partially why ZIKV infection in early pregnancy causes more serious adverse pregnancy outcomes observed in human and mouse models [12, 16, 17].

Extensive researches have focused on how ZIKV infection targeting the developing brain independently causes neurological damages in fetuses. Nonetheless, maternal ZIKV infection in human and multiple animal models resulting in microcephaly was accompanied by substantial placental insufficiency and abnormalities, where few studies keep a watchful eye on how placental structure and function are modified upon ZIKV infection and the contribution of placental defects to CZS [18, 19]. Moreover, whether ZIKV infection during pregnancy could affect neonatal development and even long-term health issues especially in those who had no obvious CZS at birth? There is evidence that some normal-appearing newborns born to the mother with ZIKV exposure during pregnancy developed a microcephaly phenotype during postnatal development, such as head growth restrictions and brain neuroimaging abnormalities. Furthermore, motor disorders and neurodevelopmental delay in the language function in infants can also be observed after birth in some ZIKV-exposed cases in utero [20]. In line with those, Paul et al. (2018) did not observe significant morphological alterations and ZIKV existence in perinatal mice after intraperitoneal ZIKV infection on pregnant dams, while manifested postnatal growth impediments and neurobehavioral deficits appeared later in postnatal life [21].

Therefore, a transient ZIKV infection during pregnancy is likely to affect future development and health of the neonates and even adulthood health in a long run, which still needs in-depth mechanistic studies to address.

Rubella infection, also known as 3-day measles or German measles (because firstly described by two German physicians), is typically mild and occurs mostly in childhood. Rubella virus (RuV) is a member of the genus Rubivirus, belonging to the family of Matonaviridae. Its genome of single-stranded RNA is enclosed by an icosahedral capsid. Transmission usually occurs through respiratory droplets but can also occur to the fetus through placenta. Vertical transmission of rubella is higher in the first weeks of gestation, leading to miscarriage, stillbirth, or a chronic injury of several organs in the fetus, well-known as Congenital rubella syndrome (CRS), includes a spectrum of several defects: eye defects (such as cataracts, microphthalmia, chorioretinitis, corneal opacity, and glaucoma), sensorineural hearing loss, cardiovascular anomalies (most commonly patent ductus arteriosus, peripheral pulmonary artery stenosis or coarctation of aorta), brain injury (like microcephaly, hydrocephalus, and cerebral calcifications) [22, 23]. Low-birth weight was observed in 9% of CRS cases [4].

During maternal viremia, RuV may cross the placental barrier and enter into the fetal circulation, causing a necrotizing vasculitis. The virus is probably transported as infected endothelial cell emboli, resulting in a chronic injury [24]. The exact mechanisms at the basis of CRS are still not completely understood, considering the near eradication of rubella and the absence of animal models to study. Gestational age at the time of maternal infection plays a key role in causing fetal damage. The risk of CRS is higher during the first 11–12 weeks of gestational age and then clearly decreases [25].

RuV antigen was detected in several organs (lung, heart, aorta and pulmonary artery, brain, placenta) of cases with a poor prognosis [25]. Apoptosis pathways have been showed to involve RuV-infected adult cells, whereas apoptosis in fetal cells was not supported and this could promote viral persistence in developing cells [26].

Furthermore, RuV infection could play an indirect role in impairing growth and differentiation mechanisms through secretion of interferon and other chemokines [27].

Chronic-induced injury has been confirmed by the observed increase of inflammatory chemokines (CCL5, CXCL10, and CXCL11) in case of RuV-infected endothelial cells. Interestingly, the chemokine CCL14 that promotes embryo implantation was down-regulated, as in parallel a set of genes involved in eye and ear development has also been shown as down-regulated in a model with RuV-infected fetal endothelial cells [28].

Maternal carriage of the hepatitis B virus during pregnancy is deemed to be an important gestational comorbidity. Congenital abnormalities, as the critical outcome susceptible to viral infection during pregnancy, are similarly possible to be affected. Based on the most comprehensive evidence, the pooling of unadjusted data in this study did not show significant association between maternal HBV infection and overall congenital abnormalities (cRR = 1.15). However, the pooling of adjusted data suggested that pregnant women with HBV infection might be associated with a higher risk of overall congenital abnormalities (aOR = 1.40). There were nearly half of the studies that did not adjust for confounders, which may be related to the low incidence of congenital abnormalities [29].

A previous meta-analysis that was published in 2015 reported no significant association between maternal HBV infection and overall congenital abnormalities (cOR = 1.10, 95% CI: 0.85–1.43; three studies included) [30]. The result in the prior study should be interpreted with caution. First, the sample size was so small that only three studies involving 1514 cases were included. The statistical power may be insufficient to detect the potential association, particularly with respect to rare events. On the other hand, the study only provided the pooled result of unadjusted data. As for an observational study, the risk of bias is always present because the allocation is non-randomized, and estimates from unadjusted data were likely to deviate from the underlying true effect [29].

The pathogenesis and etiology of congenital abnormalities induced by maternal HBV infection is poorly understood. A growing body of evidence suggests that HBV infection could increase tumor necrosis factor (TNF-α) production, which is similar to zika virus and syphilis [31–33]. Pan et al. [34] pointed out that a higher serum level TNF-α would increase the risk of congenital heart disease [34]. Furthermore, McDougall et al. [35] recently observed that HBV infection caused mitotic spindle misorientation. This anomaly may contribute, ultimately, to microcephaly [35]. In addition, HBV can be detected in non-liver tissues (lymph nodes, spleen, ovaries, and placenta) and, notably, the HBV can be transferred through the placental barrier, which may intensify subtle disorders on the fetus. Thus, more studies are encouraged to the casual effect of HBV infection on congenital abnormalities [36–38]. Specifically, the type of congenital abnormalities susceptible to HBV infection deserves increased attention.

Historically, there were attempts to explain the development of congenital malformations with other infections as well, although direct statistical proves were not acquired and appropriate genetic studies were not provided. Among these infections some data in favor of their teratogenic role was presented in herpes and mycoplasmosis. Certainly, it is impossible to exclude them, as well as other pathogens, as possible cause of congenital malformations.

Identification of factors associated with congenital anomalies has been shown to reduce treatment costs and medical complications of neonates. Therefore, genetic counseling and educational programs for high-risk women, and prenatal screening are essential to identify and prevent factors contributing to congenital abnormalities.

References

1. Ely DM, Driscoll AK. Infant mortality in the United States, 2020: data from the period linked birth/infant death file. Natl Vital Stat Rep. 2022;71(5):1–18.
2. Krauer F, Riesen M, Reveiz L, et al. Zika virus infection as a cause of congenital brain abnormalities and Guillain-Barré syndrome: systematic review. PLoS Med. 2017;14:e1002203. https://doi.org/10.1371/journal.pmed.1002203.
3. Hcini N, Kugbe Y, Rafalimanana Z, et al. Association between confirmed congenital Zika infection at birth and outcomes up to 3 years of life. Nat

Commun. 2021;12(1):3270. https://doi.org/10.1038/s41467-021-23468-3.

4. Yazigi A, De Pecoulas AE, Vauloup-Fellous C, et al. Fetal and neonatal abnormalities due to congenital rubella syndrome: a review of literature. J Matern Fetal Neonatal Med. 2017;30:274–8. https://doi.org/10.3109/14767058.2016.1169526.
5. Yu W, Hu X, Cao B. Viral infections during pregnancy: the big challenge threatening maternal and fetal health. Matern Fetal Med. 2022;4(1):72–86. https://doi.org/10.1097/FM9.0000000000000133.
6. Lowe R, Barcellos C, Brasil P, et al. The Zika virus epidemic in Brazil: from discovery to future implications. Int J Environ Res Public Health. 2018;15(1):96. https://doi.org/10.3390/ijerph15010096.
7. Adibi JJ, Marques ETA Jr, Cartus A, et al. Teratogenic effects of the Zika virus and the role of the placenta. Lancet. 2016;387(10027):1587–90. https://doi.org/10.1016/S0140-6736(16)00650-4.
8. Broxmeyer L, Kanjhan R. Does Zika really have the capacity to affect the nervous system and cause microcephaly or intracranial calcifications? Mod Res Inflamm. 2016;5(2):20–30. https://doi.org/10.4236/mri.2016.52003.
9. Microcephaly Epidemic Research Group. Microcephaly in infants, Pernambuco State, Brazil, 2015. Emerg Infect Dis. 2016;22(6):1090–3. https://doi.org/10.3201/eid2206.160062.
10. Robinson N, Mayorquin Galvan EE, Zavala Trujillo IG, et al. Congenital Zika syndrome: pitfalls in the placental barrier. Rev Med Virol. 2018;28(5):e1985. https://doi.org/10.1002/rmv.1985.
11. Li C, Xu D, Ye Q, et al. Zika virus disrupts neural progenitor development and leads to microcephaly in mice. Cell Stem Cell. 2016;19(1):120–6. https://doi.org/10.1016/j.stem.2016.04.017.
12. Chan JF, Choi GK, Yip CC, et al. Zika fever and congenital Zika syndrome: an unexpected emerging arboviral disease. J Infect. 2016;72(5):507–24. https://doi.org/10.1016/j.jinf.2016.02.011.
13. Ticconi C, Pietropolli A, Rezza G. Zika virus infection and pregnancy: what we do and do not know. Pathog Glob Health. 2016;110(7–8):262–8. https://doi.org/10.1080/20477724.2016.1234804.
14. King N, Teixeira MM, Mahalingam S. Zika virus: mechanisms of infection during pregnancy. Trends Microbiol. 2017;25(9):701–2. https://doi.org/10.1016/j.tim.2017.05.005.
15. Tan L, Lacko LA, Zhou T, et al. Pre- and peri-implantation Zika virus infection impairs fetal development by targeting trophectoderm cells. Nat Commun. 2019;10(1):4155. https://doi.org/10.1038/s41467-019-12063-2.
16. de Noronha L, Zanluca C, Burger M, et al. Zika virus infection at different pregnancy stages: anatomopathological findings, target cells and viral persistence in placental tissues. Front Microbiol. 2018;9:2266. https://doi.org/10.3389/fmicb.2018.02266.
17. Jagger BW, Miner JJ, Cao B, et al. Gestational stage and IFN-lambda signaling regulate ZIKV infection in utero. Cell Host Microbe. 2017;22(3):366–376e.3. https://doi.org/10.1016/j.chom.2017.08.012.
18. Rosenberg AZ, Yu W, Hill DA, et al. Placental pathology of Zika virus: viral infection of the placenta induces villous stromal macrophage (Hofbauer cell) proliferation and hyperplasia. Arch Pathol Lab Med. 2017;141(1):43–8. https://doi.org/10.5858/arpa.2016-0401-OA.
19. Miner JJ, Cao B, Govero J, et al. Zika virus infection during pregnancy in mice causes placental damage and fetal demise. Cell. 2016;165(5):1081–91. https://doi.org/10.1016/j.cell.2016.05.008.
20. Raper J, Chahroudi A. Clinical and preclinical evidence for adverse neurodevelopment after postnatal Zika virus infection. Trop Med Infect Dis. 2021;6(1):10. https://doi.org/10.3390/tropicalmed6010010.
21. Paul AM, Acharya D, Neupane B, et al. Congenital Zika virus infection in immunocompetent mice causes postnatal growth impediment and neurobehavioral deficits. Front Microbiol. 2018;9:2028. https://doi.org/10.3389/fmicb.2018.02028.
22. Neu N, Duchon J, Zachariah P. TORCH infections. Clin Perinatol. 2015;42:77–103. https://doi.org/10.1016/j.clp.2014.11.001.
23. Woyessa AB, Ali MS, Korkpor TK, Ii RT, Kohar HT, Dogba J, et al. Rubella transmission and the risk of congenital rubella syndrome in Liberia: a need to introduce rubella-containing vaccine in the routine immunization program. BMC Infect Dis. 2019;19:813. https://doi.org/10.1186/s12879-019-4464-7.
24. Banatvala J, Brown D. Rubella. Lancet. 2004;363:1127–37. https://doi.org/10.1016/S0140-6736(04)15897-2.
25. Lazar M, Perelygina L, Martines R, Greer P, Paddock CD, Peltecu G, et al. Immunolocalization and distribution of rubella antigen in fatal congenital rubella syndrome. EBioMedicine. 2016;3:86–92. https://doi.org/10.1016/j.ebiom.2015.11.050.
26. George S, Viswanathan R, Sapkal GN. Molecular aspects of the teratogenesis of rubella virus. Biol Res. 2019;52:1–8. https://doi.org/10.1186/s40659-019-0254-3.
27. Adamo MP, Zapata M, Frey TK. Analysis of gene expression in fetal and adult cells infected with rubella virus. Virology. 2008;370:1–11. https://doi.org/10.1016/j.virol.2007.08.003.
28. Geyer H, Bauer M, Neumann J, Lüdde A, Rennert P, Friedrich N, et al. Gene expression profiling of rubella virus infected primary endothelial cells of fetal and adult origin. Virol J. 2016;13:1–17. https://doi.org/10.1186/s12985-016-0475-9.
29. Huang S, Wang J, Xiong Y, Liu C, Qi Y, Zou K, Tan J, Sun X. Impact of maternal hepatitis B carrier status on congenital abnormalities: a systematic review and meta-analysis. BMJ Open. 2023;13(3):e066017. Published online 2023 Mar 28. https://doi.org/10.1136/bmjopen-2022-066017.
30. Luo L, Wu J, Qu Y, et al. Association between maternal HBsAg carrier status and neonatal adverse outcomes: meta-analysis. J Matern Fetal Neonatal Med.

2015;28:1308–17. https://doi.org/10.3109/14767058.2014.953475.

31. Wang H, Luo H, Wan X, et al. TNF-α/IFN-γ profile of HBV-specific CD4 T cells is associated with liver damage and viral clearance in chronic HBV infection. J Hepatol. 2020;72:45–56. https://doi.org/10.1016/j.jhep.2019.08.024.
32. Akpolat N, Yahsi S, Godekmerdan A, et al. Relationship between serum cytokine levels and histopathological changes of liver in patients with hepatitis B. World J Gastroenterol. 2005;11:3260–3. https://doi.org/10.3748/wjg.v11.i21.3260.
33. Gotlieb N, Tachlytski I, Lapidot Y, et al. Hepatitis B virus downregulates vitamin D receptor levels in hepatoma cell lines, thereby preventing vitamin D-dependent inhibition of viral transcription and production. Mol Med. 2018;24:53. https://doi.org/10.1186/s10020-018-0055-0.
34. Pan J, Hu J, Qi X, et al. Association study of a functional variant of TNF-α gene and serum TNF-α level with the susceptibility of congenital heart disease in a Chinese population. Postgrad Med J. 2019;95:547–51. https://doi.org/10.1136/postgradmedj-2019-136621.
35. McDougall WM, Perreira JM, Hung H-F, et al. Viral infection or IFN-α alters mitotic spindle orientation by modulating pericentrin levels. IScience. 2019;12:270–9. https://doi.org/10.1016/j.isci.2019.01.025.
36. Bai H, Zhang L, Ma L, et al. Relationship of hepatitis B virus infection of placental barrier and hepatitis B virus intra-uterine transmission mechanism. World J Gastroenterol. 2007;13:3625–30. https://doi.org/10.3748/wjg.v13.i26.3625.
37. Yoffe B, Burns DK, Bhatt HS, et al. Extrahepatic hepatitis B virus DNA sequences in patients with acute hepatitis B infection. Hepatology. 1990;12:187–92. https://doi.org/10.1002/hep.1840120202.
38. Datta S. Compartmentalization of hepatitis B virus: looking beyond the liver. World J Hepatol. 2015;7:2241–4. https://doi.org/10.4254/wjh.v7.i20.2241.

9 Clinical Manifestations of Intrauterine Infections

9.1 Children with Mild Intrauterine Infectious Pathology

In the conditions of a physiological maternity hospital, a comprehensive clinical, laboratory, and morphological study of women in labor, afterbirth, and newborn children was conducted, aimed at detecting herpes, mycoplasmosis, chlamydia, and cytomegaly using modern enzyme immunoassay, serological, immunofluorescence, cytological, and histological methods was provided in collaboration with NM Bogdanova. Infant's catamnesis was traced for 18 months. It was shown that 75.7% of the examined women in labor had a history of inflammatory diseases of the genitals after abortions, which contributed to the pathological course of pregnancy.

It was found that pregnant women have a high incidence of somatic (60.4%), gynecological (59.4%), urological (61.3%) pathology and anemia (63.9%). The course of pregnancy is most often disrupted by pathological weight gain (62.3%) and the threat of miscarriage (52.2%). The relationship of the pathological course of childbirth and pregnancy with infection has been statistically confirmed. It has been shown that cervical erosion, endometritis, ovarian dysfunction, stillbirth, spontaneous miscarriage, pathological course of labor (in anamnesis), leukocyturia, pyelonephritis, threat of termination of pregnancy, weakness of labor, development of preeclampsia in childbirth occurs more often in women infected with *M. hominis* and/or *C. trachomatis*.

In any form, localization and etiology of the infectious process, placentitis develops in the pregnant woman (99.1%), accompanied by a violation of barrier function, in the form of subcompensated (42.3%) and decompensated (10.8%) placental insufficiency. In 70.3% of the cases, the etiology of placentas was mixed.

It has been shown that when all the membranes of the afterbirth are affected, intrauterine infection of the fetus occurs in 46.8% of cases. The most contagious pathogen affecting the fetus in 84.2% of cases is chlamydia.

When analyzing medical documentation, it was found that the predisposing factor of antenatal infection is complicated medical abortion ($p < 0.01$). The complicated course of the intranatal period was more often observed in the group of seropositive children with a pronounced degree of placental insufficiency. It was found that weakness of labor activity develops more often in women at birth of an antenatally infected fetus ($p < 0.01$). The pathological course of the early neonatal period was more often noted in the group of seropositive children and manifested by purulent conjunctivitis, dyspeptic and bronchopulmonary disorders, liver damage ($p < 0.05$–0.01).

Neurological symptoms were noted in 92.3% of seropositive and 83.0% of seronegative

V. Zinserling et al., *Placentitis and Perinatal Infections*,
https://doi.org/10.1007/978-3-031-80553-0_9

children born with impaired compensatory functions of the placenta, especially with acute decompensation. Hypoxic-ischemic lesions of the cerebral cortex lead to impaired differentiation and synthesis, which is manifested by a decrease in fine motor skills, diffuse muscular hypotension, single elements of pyramidal insufficiency, speech delay. During dynamic monitoring of children, it was found that by the year, due to high neuroplasticity, it is possible to stop the pronounced neurological symptoms that arose as a result of damage to the centers of the thalamo-pallidar system. In the seronegative group, the recovery process is faster.

The incidence of acute respiratory diseases in the seropositive group in the first year and a half was higher than in the seronegative group. The peak of colds occurs during the period of 6–9 months in both groups. The number of hospitalizations in the seropositive group aged 3 months and 7–11 months was 2.5–3 times higher than in the seronegative group. The course of acute respiratory infections in seropositive children was protracted with the development of complications in the form of bronchitis, pneumonia, and otitis media. It was found that acute respiratory infections in the first year of life were more likely to develop in children who had suffered acute or chronic hypoxia associated with placental insufficiency.

The frequency of harmonious physical development in the group of seropositive children was also lower than in the group of seronegative children.

Thus, using this material, it was possible to prove that intrauterine infection very often occurs even with relatively favorable clinical and laboratory indicators. It is very important to notice that, on the one hand, intrauterine infection can significantly affect various organs and systems of the child, including (especially in the case of central nervous system damage) with late manifestation. On the other hand, it is important to remember that intrauterine infections are by no means fatal diseases and, with a favorable combination of circumstances, complete self-healing is possible. The condition of the afterbirth, associated with the compensatory and adaptive capabilities of the child, also has a significant impact on the prognosis for intrauterine infections.

9.2 Low-Grade Intrauterine Infections in Pediatric Patients with Central Nervous System Diseases

In collaboration with Yu.I. Weinshenker, 42 pediatric patients with chronic neurological diseases were examined: 3–7 years old—22 patients, 8–11 years old—8, 12–15 years old—12. Girls—17, boys—25.

Searches were conducted for chlamydia, mycoplasmas, ureaplasma, pathogenic capsular bacteroids. Cerebrospinal fluid, blood, flushes, and scrapings from mucous membranes were examined in 13 people, blood and mucous membranes in the remaining 29. Methods: cultural, PCR, serological.

In 88% (37/42 patients), these are infectious pathogens have been identified in various combinations. No pathogens were found in the remaining patients.

Chlamydia was detected in 30/42 (71%) patients. As a monoinfection (with various combinations of *C. trachomatis*, *C. pneumoniae*, *C. psittaci*)—in 8 out of 30 patients: in cerebrospinal fluid—in 6/13 (46%) (in 2—only in cerebrospinal fluid / periodically cerebrospinal fluid and nasopharynx, in 2—in cerebrospinal fluid and blood, in 2—in cerebrospinal fluid, blood and nasopharynx/genital (periodically only in the cerebrospinal fluid and nasopharynx)), in the blood—in 18/42, In the nasopharynx—in 21/42, genital—7/9.

In 27/30 of the observations, chlamydia was detected culturally and/or by PCR, while 8 of these patients (out of 27) had no antibodies to chlamydia infection (!). In 3/30 of the observations (in all cases, cerebrospinal fluid was not studied), only antibodies were detected, and the bacteria themselves were not detected: in 2/3—at to *C. trachomatis*, 1/3—*C. pneumoniae* + *C. psittaci*.

Mycoplasma was found in 13/42 (31%) patients. As a monoinfection: in 1/13 primary; in

4/13 patients—in the long-term period after rehabilitation from chlamydia.

In the cerebrospinal fluid of 3/13 (in 2—in the cerebrospinal fluid, blood and nasopharynx, in 1—in the cerebrospinal fluid and blood); in the blood of 6/42, in the nasopharynx of 8/42, genital—2/9.

Ureaplasma was found in 6/42 (14%) patients. As a monoinfection—in 1. In the cerebrospinal fluid—it was not detected, in the blood—in 3/42, in the nasopharynx—at 4/42, genital—not detected.

Bacteroides fragilis was found in 21/42 (50%) patients as monoinfection B. fr. was found in two patients without cerebrospinal fluid examination.

In the cerebrospinal fluid—in 6/13 (in 1—in the cerebrospinal fluid, in 2—in the cerebrospinal fluid and nasopharynx, in 3—in the cerebrospinal fluid, blood, and nasopharynx).

In the blood—in 9/42 (in 3—in the cerebrospinal fluid, blood, and nasopharynx, in the remaining six patients, the cerebrospinal fluid was not examined and the pathogen was determined only in the blood (in 2) and in the blood and nasopharynx (4)).

In the nasopharynx—in 18/42 (in 9—only in the nose, but patients without puncture).

The data provided by our studies of various years, performed using various methods, clearly indicate a significant frequency of intrauterine infections, especially perinatal chlamydiosis. Various pathogens from this group can play an etiological role in the development of pathology of pregnancy, fetus, newborn, and older children. The nature of the clinical manifestations of the disease can vary significantly from practically asymptomatic to fatal, with the most characteristic being the chronic course. Morphological changes in chlamydiosis of different localizations are similar, although they are little known and can be used in diagnosis. Many issues related to the epidemiology, pathogenesis, and morphological manifestations of intrauterine infections need further study.

Conclusion

Intrauterine infections are currently one of the leading pathologies of childhood worldwide, primarily in developing countries. They not only lead to a high mortality rate, especially in the perinatal period, but also in some cases cause profound disability due to congenital malformations and chronic diseases.

Numerous studies indicate the important role of intrauterine infections, but there are practically no works on their morphological diagnosis and frequency on autopsy material.

The increasing frequency of infection of a pregnant woman in modern conditions makes this problem relevant. The nature of the immune restructuring of her body gives originality to the course of the infectious process during pregnancy. It is likely that as a result of this, prerequisites are created for a more pronounced than usual generalization of infection and the entry of pathogens into the afterbirth.

The lesion of the afterbirth can be caused by all known classes of microorganisms. However, viral, mycoplasmal, and chlamydial placentitis are currently almost unexplored. There is no data on the features of inflammatory changes depending on the class of biological pathogens. Examination of the afterbirth is necessary to determine the nature of the infectious process in the mother—placenta—amniotic fluid—fetus system; however, a systematic approach is not used. In the case of antenatal fetal death, the afterbirth becomes the most important source of information for diagnosis and determination of the cause of death.

The boundaries of the use of the term "placentitis" and the principles of its differentiation from the morphological manifestations of protective reactions of the placenta remain debatable. In most of the nosologies we studied, the lesions were accompanied by the formation of antibodies in the child's blood, retroplacental blood, and amniotic fluid with a four-fold or more excess compared to their titers in the maternal blood. In these afterbirths, along with characteristic structural changes, antigens of pathogens (viruses and mycoplasmas), as well as cellular inflammatory reactions, were detected. All this made it possible to consider such lesions as placentitis, despite the absence of significant cellular infiltration in them.

It should also be noted that not every lesion of the afterbirth is accompanied by the development of an intrauterine infection. Most babies are born on time, viable, and even healthy. Therefore, it is very important to study its compensatory reactions, protective functions, including specific immune ones. It should be noted that there is insufficient data on this issue, and morphological work is almost completely absent. Finally, determining the nature of the lesions of the afterbirth allows in some cases to identify a chronic infection of the mother as well as predict a tendency to infectious and some other diseases caused by respiratory viruses, viruses from the herpes group, mycoplasmas and chlamydia.

For many years, we have been conducting a comprehensive study of infectious lesions, according to the principles developed by A. V. Zinserling, using morphological and virological

V. Zinserling et al., *Placentitis and Perinatal Infections*, https://doi.org/10.1007/978-3-031-80553-0

methods in combination with the identification of pathogens and their antigens in affected tissues and the determination of antibodies to these pathogens. It should be noted that the analysis of significant materials using a variety of methods (light, electron, IF microscopy, immunohistochemistry, virus isolation, serological studies, computer analysis) has not been conducted by anyone in the world before.

Currently, different points of view are expressed in the literature on the reliability of the etiological verification of the process. It is often said that the use of modern molecular biological methods (PCR, in situ hybridization) is mandatory. Our experience allows us to state with full confidence that obtaining consistent results using at least two traditional methods (histology, IF microscopy, serology) gives reliable results. Histological and cytological methods (of course, when carried out by qualified specialists) give, especially during screening studies, quite reliable results. However, the isolated use of only one molecular biological method (for example, high-quality PCR for the diagnosis of cytomegaly) can lead to overdiagnosis. Many authors agree that PCR research in chlamydia infection can give false negative results, there are no explanations for this phenomenon in the literature.

This manual contains and systematizes the results of many years of research conducted by pathologists specialized in infections in St. Petersburg, which made it possible for the first time in the world literature to give a complete morphological characterization of lesions of the afterbirth and fetus by many pathogens. Unfortunately, we were not able to systematically identify all possible etiological factors of perinatal infections. In the initial period of research, this applies to chlamydia and hepatitis. For a long time, lesions caused by entero- and parvoviruses have not been diagnosed in our material. One can only assume their role in terms of observations, especially in mixed infections. Currently, very relevant lesions caused by human immunodeficiency viruses and new coronaviruses have been studied in depth only on limited material.

Placentitis caused by mycoplasmas were found on our materials from previous years. Considering that a new species of mycoplasma has now been discovered—*M. genitalium*, which has a number of antigens in common with *M. pneumoniae*, we assume that the lesions caused by these two pathogens are indistinguishable. It should be noted that the described changes fully corresponded to the descriptions of lesions in mycoplasmosis in other organs.

In recent years, our team has studied in detail the morphological manifestations of placentitis caused by chlamydia, hepatitis viruses, HIV, and the new coronavirus. For the first time in the world literature, on the basis of extensive clinical, laboratory, and morphological comparisons, the features of structural changes in the afterbirth in these infections are shown, allowing, with sufficient experience, to roughly determine the etiology of the process. It should be noted that the accuracy of the data obtained has been repeatedly verified by us both through expert revisions of laboratory-confirmed observations and using IHC. At the same time, it should be noted that a number of details concerning the peculiarities of the relationship between pathogens and the cellular systems of the afterbirth require further study.

Chlamydia, according to both literature and own data, is a fairly common infection in both children and adults. Despite the significant amount of work devoted to some aspects of this problem in recent years, many topical issues remain almost unexplored. Our data indicate the reliability of the well-known principles of cytological and histological diagnostics based on rather specific microscopic changes. We do not share the opinion of a number of authors about the low sensitivity of the morphological method. The results of the comparison of morphological and laboratory data confirm the sufficient reliability of the histological and cytological investigation. Chlamydia infection according our experience can vary in a very wide range of severity, which, of course, depends on the state of immunity and local reactivity of the mucous membranes, and very likely on the individual properties of the pathogen.

Recently, we got the opportunity to study the lesions of the afterbirth caused by the human immunodeficiency virus and the new coronavirus.

Placentitis caused by other pathogens: rubella viruses, measles, chickenpox, Mycobacterium tuberculosis, pale treponema, listeria were studied by us on relatively limited material. The nature of the revealed structural changes generally corresponded to the literature data.

It has been established that in a significant part of cases, placentitis are caused by several pathogens (viruses and mycoplasmas). Among the pathogens that are more common in mixed infections of the afterbirth, influenza viruses, herpes simplex and mycoplasma and chlamydia should be noted. This is due to the highest prevalence of these infections among the population, either in manifest form, like influenza, or inapparant form, like herpes or mycoplasmosis.

When analyzing the materials of recent years, there is also a significant frequency in the composition of mixed placentas with the participation of chlamydial lesions.

In the presence of infection in the mother—placenta-fetus system, the afterbirth is the central link, and in relation to the fetus, a barrier to exogenous infection of the embryo. The facts of intrauterine fetal infection are widely known in the literature; however, its mechanism has not been sufficiently studied. The claim of transplacental transmission of infection is often not supported by the data of morphological examination of the afterbirth. In this regard, it is widely believed that the pathogen can penetrate into the fetus through an unchanged placenta. This fact is also explained by the fact that non-specific changes in the afterbirth occur a second time, most often as a result of impaired blood circulation and metabolic processes. They are much more pronounced than those lesions that occur when infected with pathogens that multiply intracellularly.

There are also facts about the presence of antibodies to pathogens in the fetus, and their level can significantly exceed the level of antibodies in the mother's blood. However, the place of antibody production is still the subject of discussion. There are three points of view: (1) antibodies are transmitted through the placenta from the mother, (2) they are produced by the fetus itself, (3) the production of antibodies by the placenta is possible.

Based on the results we obtained in previous years, it can be assumed that antibodies can be produced by the placenta itself. This position is supported by the presence in a number of observations of higher antibody titers in retroplacental blood compared with their levels in the mother and fetus.

With the flow of maternal blood, the pathogen appears in the intervillous space and penetrates into the syncytiotrophoblast, where its replication takes place. Due to the fact that syncytiotrophoblast is a multi-nucleus long-lived formation replenished by cytotrophoblast at the sites of damage, the pathogen (virus, mycoplasma) can accumulate in significant quantities. Thus, by comparing the structural changes in the afterbirth, the presence of lymphocytic infiltrates and vertical seroconversion in it, as well as pathogen antigens and fuchsinophilic inclusions, only those observations where there is a combination of all these signs can be considered placentitis. In the absence of all these components of the inflammatory reaction, we consider it correct to use the term "infection of the afterbirth." It should be noted that, according to our data, infection of the afterbirth is very frequent.

Along with structural changes in the afterbirth caused by direct exposure to pathogens, significant non-specific changes were found, which, first of all, were characterized by damage to the vascular bed of the villi. They were associated with a violation of placental or uteroplacental circulation. At the same time, complex dynamic processes develop in the placenta, some of which can be considered as a manifestation of insufficiency, and others as compensatory and adaptive.

Despite the fact that the concept of morphofunctional insufficiency of the placenta has been studied quite fully in non-infectious pathology, detailed systematic data on infectious placentas are practically absent. Manifestations of placental insufficiency include the presence of vascular villi, and signs of compensation include their vascularization, the presence of syncytiocapillary membranes in the villi, the formation of syncytial nodes and Langhans cells.

It should be noted that our materials for the first time prove the existence of not only severe and extremely severe forms of intrauterine infections, but also much more frequent moderate and mild ones, which in the structure of the diagnosis may be in the category of concomitant diseases. Currently, there is a variety of irrefutable evidence of a significant effect of intrauterine infection on the development of a child, including the formation of various lesions of the central nervous system in children of different ages and chronic respiratory pathology. However, many aspects of this complex problem require further study.

Infection with chlamydia, mycoplasmas, genital herpes viruses, and other pathogens in adults in many cases is certainly associated with sexual infection, but activation of a long-term chronic perinatal infection cannot be excluded.

Concluding this book, it should be noted that infectious lesions of the afterbirth in modern conditions are a common form of pathology with characteristic morphological manifestations that significantly affect the course of pregnancy, childbirth, fetal development, and postnatal diseases of the child. Morphological examination of placentas should be included in the complex of diagnostics of intrauterine infections in order to retrospectively assess the infection of a pregnant woman and determine the prognosis for the child.

GPSR Compliance

The European Union's (EU) General Product Safety Regulation (GPSR) is a set of rules that requires consumer products to be safe and our obligations to ensure this.

If you have any concerns about our products, you can contact us on ProductSafety@springernature.com

In case Publisher is established outside the EU, the EU authorized representative is:

Springer Nature Customer Service Center GmbH
Europaplatz 3
69115 Heidelberg, Germany

Batch number: 10745899

Printed by Printforce, the Netherlands